Comprehensive Computer Learning

Microsoft
Excel 2010

I0104047

Bittu Kumar

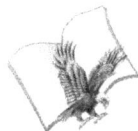

V&S PUBLISHERS

Published by:

V&S PUBLISHERS

F-2/16, Ansari road, Daryaganj, New Delhi-110002
☎ 23240026, 23240027 • *Fax:* 011-23240028
Email: info@vspublishers.com • *Website:* www.vspublishers.com

Regional Office : Hyderabad
5-1-707/1, Brij Bhawan (Beside Central Bank of India Lane)
Bank Street, Koti, Hyderabad - 500 095
☎ 040-24737290
E-mail: vspublishershyd@gmail.com

Branch Office : Mumbai
Jaywant Industrial Estate, 1st Floor–108, Tardeo Road
Opposite Sobo Central Mall, Mumbai – 400 034
☎ 022-23510736
E-mail: vspublishersmum@gmail.com

Follow us on: t f in

Printed at Repro Knowledgecast Limited, Thane

Publisher's Note

After successfully publishing youth-oriented books and getting commendable appreciation from students, teachers and parents alike, V&S Publishers is venturing into the arena of student and job-oriented books with a series of computer books on various important subjects for readers of all ages. Written and presented in lucid language and simple terms, without any computer jargon, these books are an easy-to-follow manual for readers. For the convenience of readers the information is set out in an easy to understand, step-by-step format, with clear illustrations and detailed explanations to accompany each action.

Today we live in a world of computers. The present scenario is that computers are used in every field be it education, business, trade and commerce, home and hobby, or even our ordinary day-to-day life. The importance of computers is an undeniable fact in today's world. In fact, we can't think of a world without computers.

Realising this indisputable fact, we are coming up with the series of **"Comprehensive Computer Learning (CCL)"** books. The series currently includes –

1. Comprehensive Computer Learning (CCL)
2. Comprehensive Computer Learning – A Youngsters' Guide
3. Comprehensive Computer Learning – Microsoft Office 2010
4. Comprehensive Computer Learning – Desktop Publishing (DTP)
5. Comprehensive Computer Learning – Adobe Photoshop
6. Comprehensive Computer Learning – Microsoft Excel 2010
7. Comprehensive Computer Learning – Word 2010
8. Comprehensive Computer Learning – PowerPoint 2010
9. Comprehensive Computer Learning – Publisher, Access & Outlook 210

Key features of these books:

- ❏ Written in simple and lucid language
- ❏ Presented in step-by-step, easy-to-understand format with detailed explanations with appropriate images & screenshots, charts & tables
- ❏ Useful tips and notes given in every chapter as additional information

This book **"Comprehensive Computer Learning – Microsoft Excel 2010"** has been written keeping in mind the needs of layman. MS Office & Excel with its new look & real in its 2010 version is becoming more popular at offices & home and the book explains the basics of the same in some detail.

While every effort has been made to minimise printing and other errors, it may be possible that a few might have managed to escape the wakeful eyes. We would like to request the readers to bring these errors to our notice so that we can rectify the same in subsequent editions.

Preface

This book is for the users of Microsoft Excel 2010 who want to learn the program without wasting time and efforts. Look in this book to find out how you can get your work done better and faster with these programs. Here we will discuss basic and advanced concepts of MS Excel.

What Makes this Book Different

You are holding in your hands a computer book designed to make mastering the Microsoft Excel as easy and comfortable as possible. Besides the fact that this book is easy to read, it's different from other books about Office. Read on to see why.

What do you need

❑ Latest Edition of Microsoft Excel 2010

❑ Windows operating system: All people who have the Windows operating system installed on their computers are invited to read this book. It serves for people who have Windows 7, Windows Vista, Windows XP, and Windows NT.

❑ Basic Knowledge of English

What will you get

After a comprehensive reading of this book you will be able to do a variety of jobs. And you will notice that now you can do office-related works also.

– Bittu Kumar

Contents

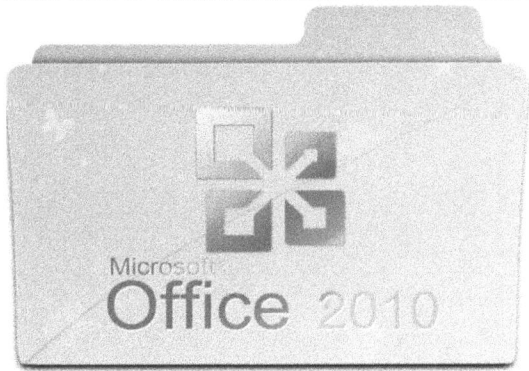

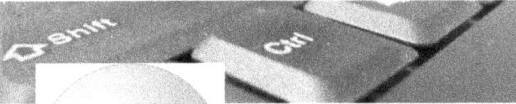

Installing MS Office 2010

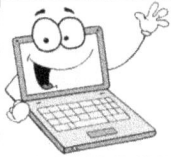

this Chapter you will learn

- How to Install Microsoft-Office 2010 on your Computer.
- Step-by-step guide of installing Microsoft Office 2010 on your Computer.

The Most Important thing is installing the Microsoft Office on your Systems First. You can do it by purchasing a genuine copy of Microsoft Office from nearest software outlet, or simply download it from the Microsoft's official website. Here we are discussing setup instructions for Microsoft Office Professional Plus 2010.

After buying CD/Downloading files, follow these Instructions:

✓ Go to the File directory where the Microsoft office setup is.

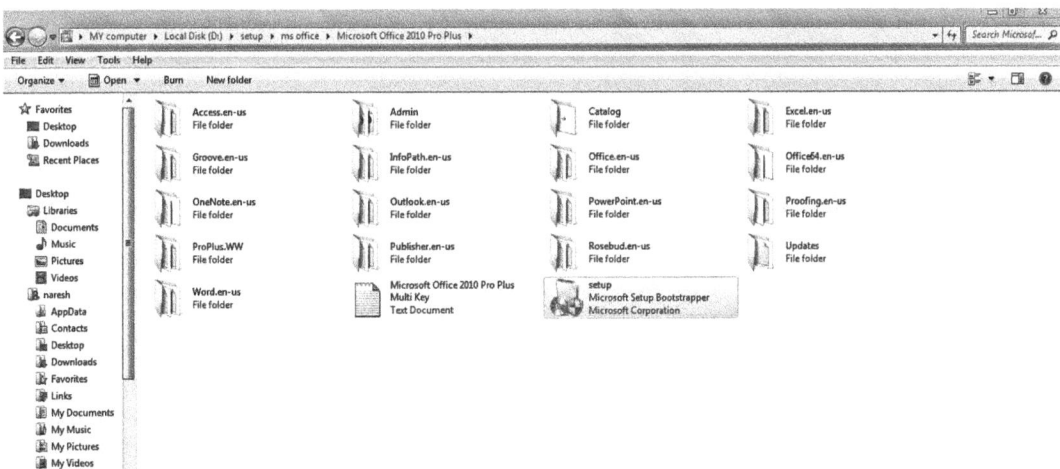

✓ Now click on Setup.exe and click on yes (In the case you are using Windows 7 or Vista).

✓ After sometime, the following dialog box will appear on your computer, Click "Install Now".

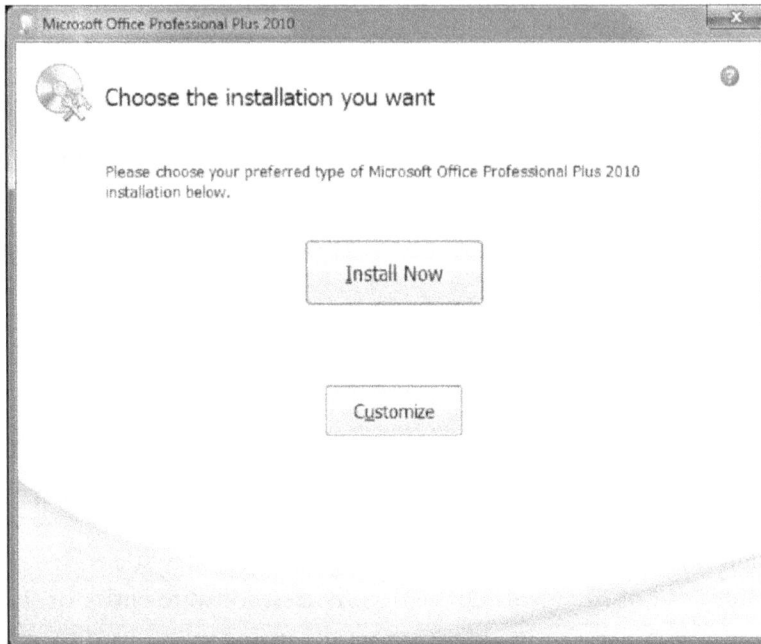

✓ The following box will appear on clicking "Install Now", wait for a few minutes and let Microsoft office 2011 be installed on your system.

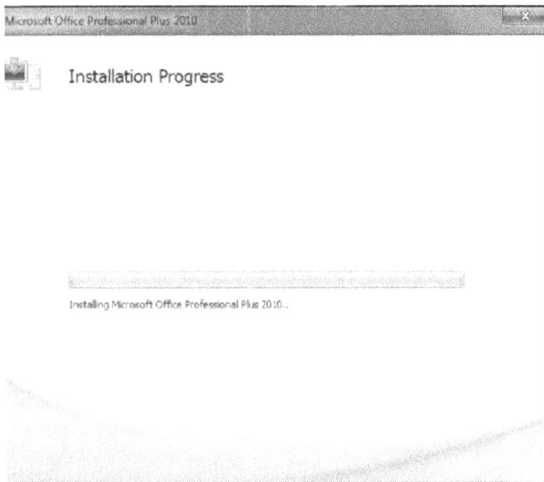

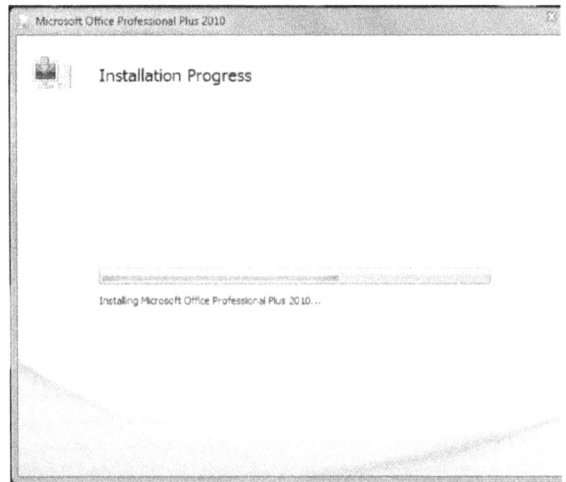

✓ Then Click "Close" and Cheers; you are done!

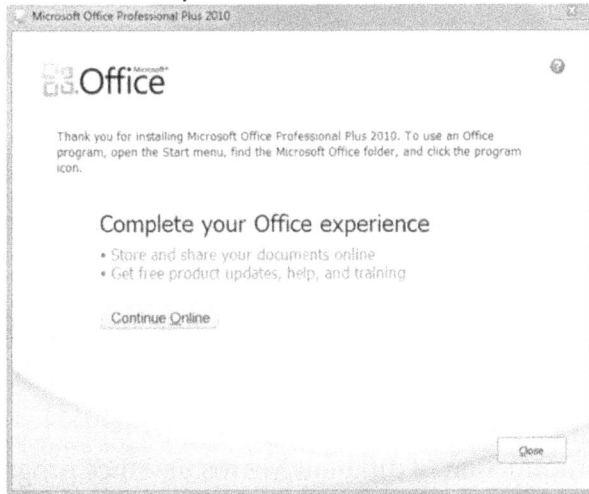

Now you have successfully Installed Microsoft office 2010 on your Computer. Now we shall begin Microsoft Office 2010 Basic Course

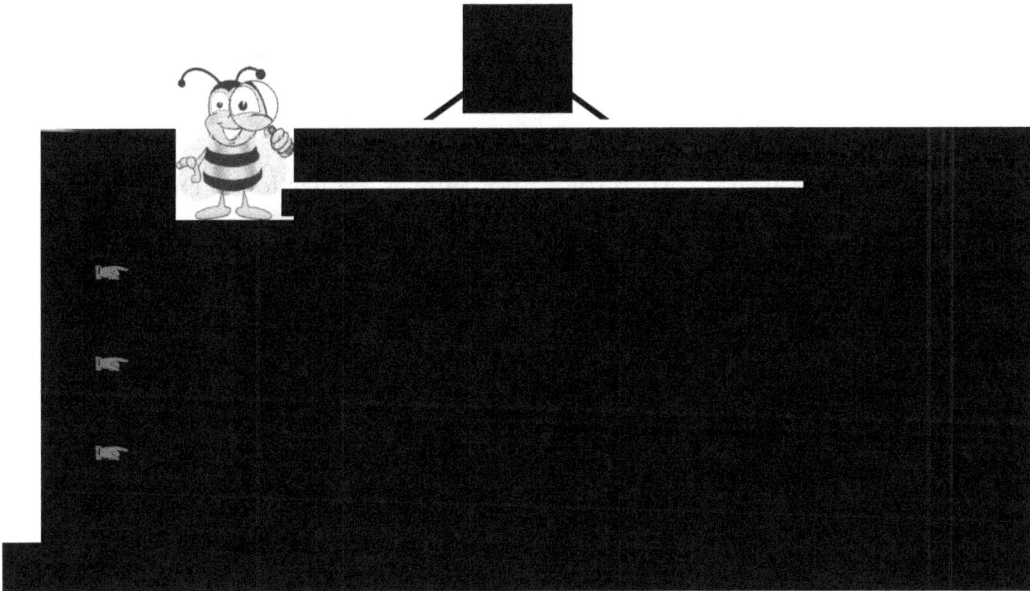

Introduction to MS Office

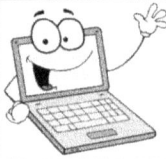

this chapter you will learn

- Introduction to different Microsoft Office programs
- Basic Information on the Graphical-User Interference
- Using different tabs in office Programs
- Creating, Saving & Editing your work
- Saving File in the earlier versions of Microsoft Office
- Encrypting the documents

Office 2010, sometimes called the Microsoft Office Suite, is a collection of computer programs. Why is it called Office? I think, because the people who developed it wanted to make software for completing tasks that need doing in a typical office. When you hear someone talk about "Office" or the "Office Software," they're talking about several different programs:

❑ **Word:** A word processor for writing letters, reports, and so on. A Word file is called a document.

❑ **Outlook:** A personal information manager, scheduler, and e-mailer.

❑ **PowerPoint:** A means of creating slide presentations to give in front of audiences. A PowerPoint file is called a presentation, or sometimes a slide show.

❑ **Excel:** A Part of office for performing numerical analyses. An Excel file is called a workbook.

❑ **Access:** A database management program.

❑ **Publisher:** A means of creating desktop-publishing files — pamphlets, notices, newsletters, and even books!

If you're new to Office, don't study so many different computer programs. The programs have much in common. You find the same commands throughout Office. For example, the method of choosing fonts is the same in Word, Outlook, PowerPoint, Excel, Access, and Publisher. Creating diagrams and charts works the same way in Word, PowerPoint, and Excel.

Starting an Office Program

Unless you start an Office program, you can't create a document, construct a worksheet, or make a database. Learn how you can do that.

✓ Click the Start button, choose All Programs → Microsoft Office, and then choose the program's name on the submenu.

User Interface in Microsoft Office

Interface, also called the user interface, is a computer term that describes how a software program presents itself to the people who use it.

Introduction to the GUI

❑ File tab

In the upper-left corner of the window is the File tab, Go to the File tab to find commands for creating, opening, and saving files, as well as doing other file-management tasks. Notice

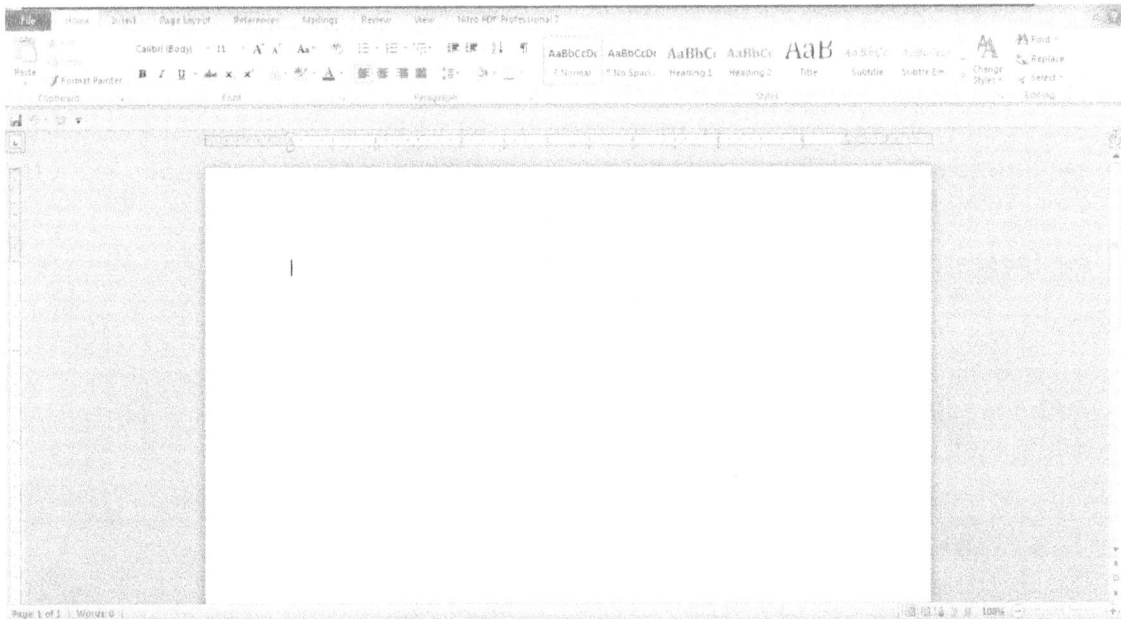

the Options command. You can choose Options to open the Options dialog box and tell the program you are working in how you want it to work.

The Ribbon and its tabs

Across the top of the screen is the Ribbon, an assortment of different tabs; click a tab to undertake a task. For example, click the Home tab to format text; click the Insert tab to insert a table or chart.

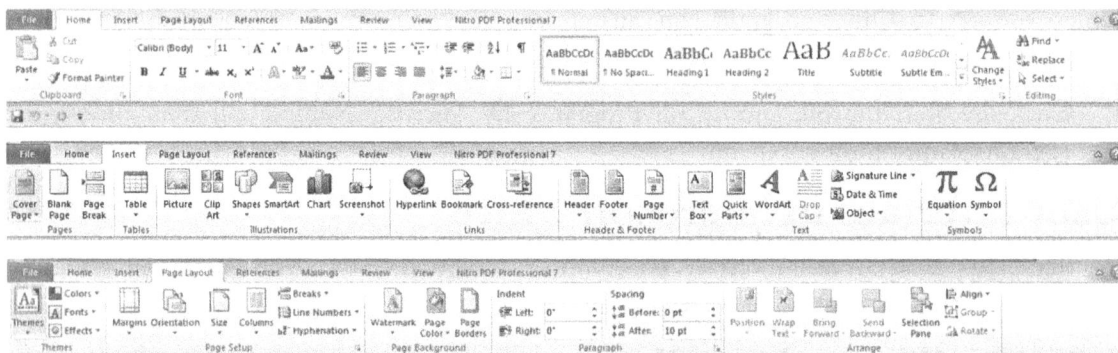

Your first step when you start a new task is to click a tab on the Ribbon. Knowing which tab to click takes a while, but the names of tabs — Home, Insert, View, and so on — hint as to which commands you find while you visit a tab.

To make the Ribbon disappear and get more room to view items on-screen, click the Minimize the Ribbon button (or press Ctrl+F1). This button is located on the right side of the Ribbon, to the left of the Help button. You can also right-click the Ribbon and choose Minimize the Ribbon on the shortcut menu, or double-click a tab on the Ribbon. To see the Ribbon again, click the Minimize the Ribbon button, press Ctrl+F1, double-click a Ribbon tab or right-click a tab name or the Quick Access toolbar and deselect Minimize the Ribbon on the shortcut menu. While the Ribbon is minimized, you can click a tab name to display a tab.

The Description of a tab

Groups

Commands on each tab are organized into groups. The names of these groups appear below the buttons and galleries on tabs. For example, the Home tab in Word is organized into several groups, including the Clipboard, Font, Paragraph, Styles.

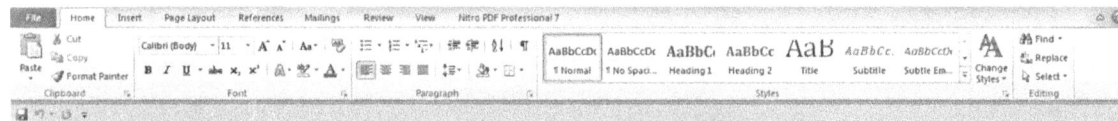

Groups do the following:

❑ Groups tell you what the buttons and galleries above their names are used for. On the Home tab in Word, for example, the buttons in the Font group are for formatting text. Read group names to help find the command you need.

❑ Many groups have a group button that you can click to open a dialog box or task pane (officially, Microsoft calls these little buttons dialog launcher).

Buttons

Go to any tab and you find buttons of all shapes and sizes. Square buttons and rectangular buttons; big and small buttons, buttons with labels and buttons without labels. Is there any rhyme or reason to these button shapes and sizes? No, there isn't. What matters isn't a button's shape or size, but whether a down-pointingarrow appears on its face:

❑ A button with an arrow: Click a button with an arrow and you get a drop-down list with options you can select.

❑ A button without an arrow: Click a button without an arrow and you complete an action of some kind.

❑ A hybrid button with an arrow: Some buttons serve a dual purpose as a button and a drop-down list. By clicking the symbol on the top half of the button, you complete an action; by clicking the arrow on the bottom half of the button, you open a drop-down list. On the Home tab, for example, clicking the top half of the Paste button pastes what is on the Clipboard into your file, but clicking the bottom half of the button opens a drop-down list with Paste options.

Keyboard Shortcuts

People who like to give commands by pressing keyboard shortcuts may well ask, "Is there keyboard shortcuts in Office?" The answer is: Yes, Office has shortcuts. For example, you can press Ctrl+B to boldface text and Ctrl+U tounderline text. Office offers Alt+key shortcuts as well.

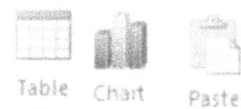

Table   Chart   Paste

Saving Your Files

Soon after you create a file, be sure to save it. And save your file from time to time while you work on it as well. Until you save your work, it rests in the computer's electronic memory (Random Access Memory), a precarious location. If a power outage occurs, you may lose all the work you did since the last time you saved your file. Make it a habit to save files every five Minutes or so or when you are doing an important task. Choose the folder where you want to save a file, declare where you want to save files by default, save files for use in 97–2003 editions of Office, and handle files that were saved automatically after a computer failure.

To save a file:

✓ Click the Save button (you find it on the Quick Access toolbar).

✓ Press Ctrl+S.

✓ Go to the File tab and choose Save.

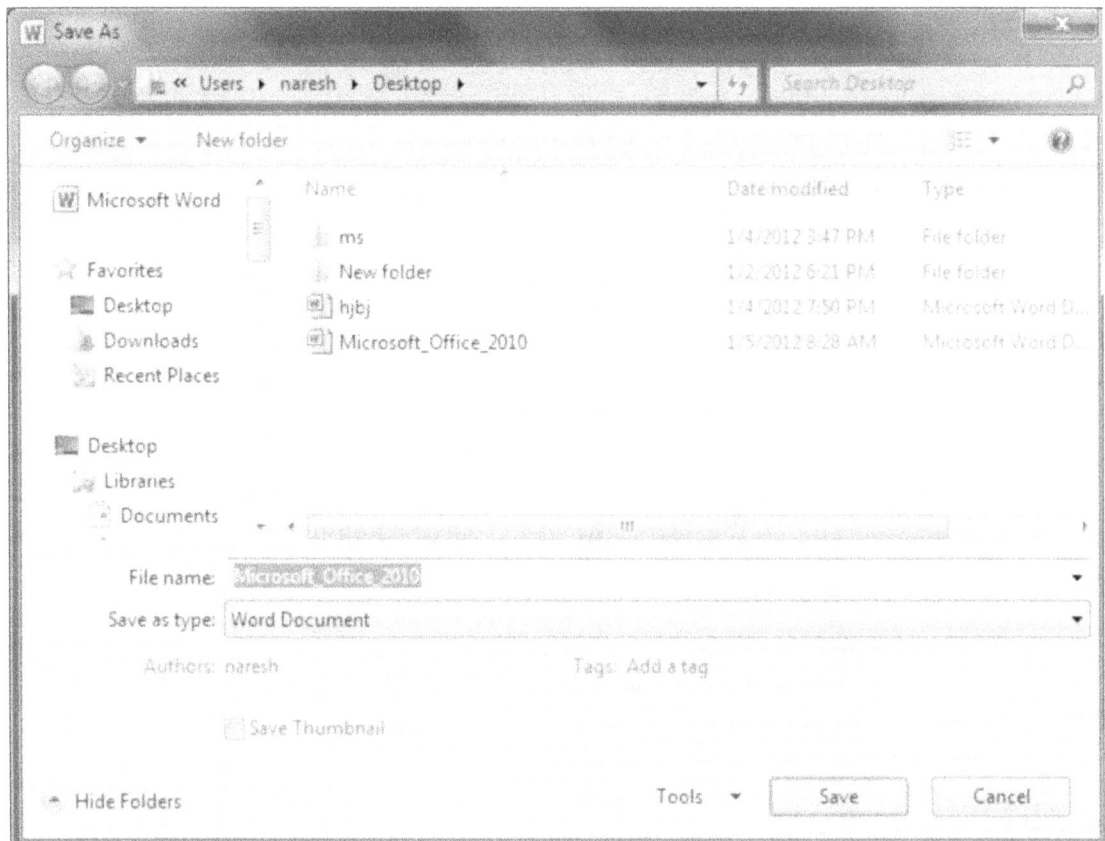

Where you like to save files

To direct Office to the folder you like best and make it appear first in the Save As and Open dialog boxes, follow these steps:

✓ In Word, Excel, PowerPoint, or Access, go to the File tab and choose Options.

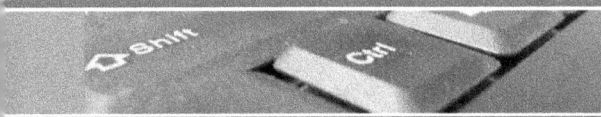

You see the Options dialog box.

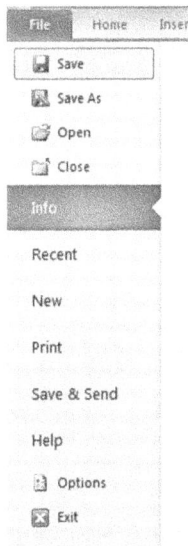

File   Home   Insert

- Save
- Save As
- Open
- Close

Info

Recent

New

Print

Save & Send

Help

Options

Exit

✓ In Word, Excel, and PowerPoint, select the Save category; in Access, select the General category.

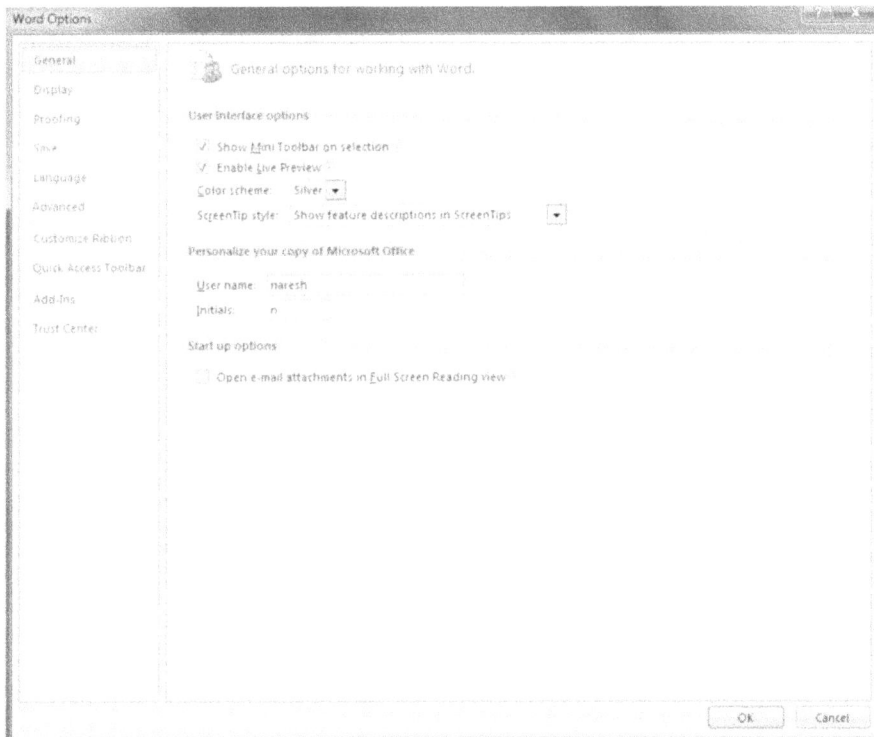

Word Options

General

Display

Proofing

Save

Language

Advanced

Customize Ribbon

Quick Access Toolbar

Add-Ins

Trust Center

General options for working with Word.

User Interface options

✓ Show Mini Toolbar on selection
✓ Enable Live Preview
Color scheme: Silver ▾
ScreenTip style: Show feature descriptions in ScreenTips ▾

Personalize your copy of Microsoft Office

User name: naresh
Initials: n

Start up options

☐ Open e-mail attachments in Full Screen Reading view

OK   Cancel

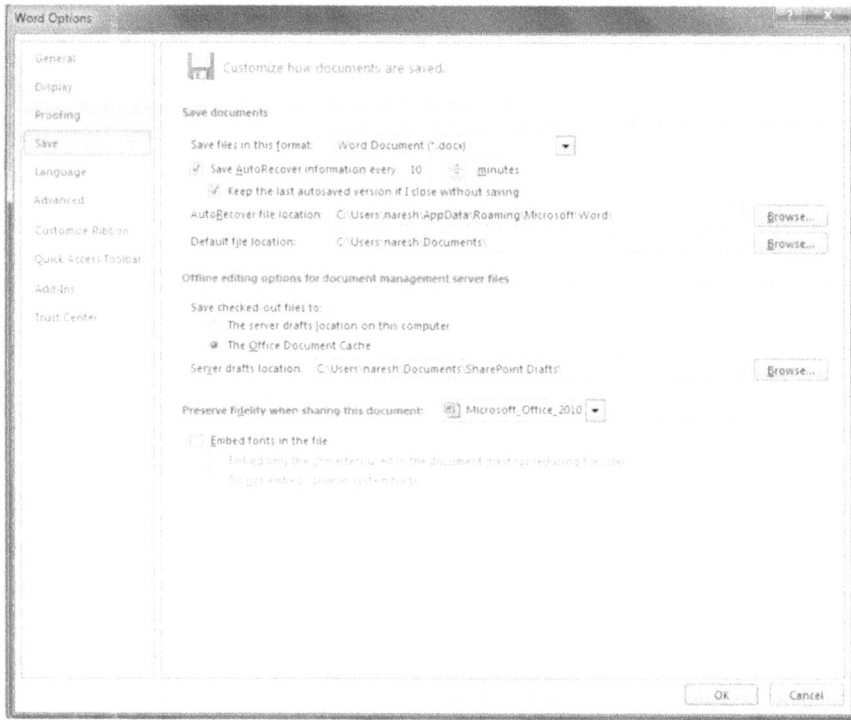

Saving a file in word

Saving files for use in earlier versions of an Office program

Before you pass along a file to a user who has Office 2003, XP, 2000, or 97, save your document in these versions so that the other person can open it. People with versions of Office prior to version 2010 and 2007 cannot open your Office files unless you save your files for earlier versions of Office.

Program	2010, 2007	97–2003
Access	.accdb	.mlb
Excel	.xlsx	.xls
PowerPoint	.pptx	.ppt
Publisher	.pub	.pub
Word	.docx	.doc

Saving a file for use in Office 97–2003

Follow these steps to save a file so that someone with Office 97, 2000, XP, or2003 can open it:

✓ Go to the File tab.

✓ Choose Save & Send.

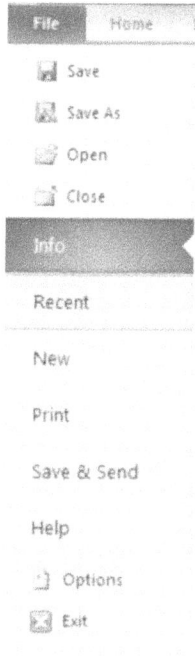

File | Home

- Save
- Save As
- Open
- Close

Info

Recent

New

Print

Save & Send

Help

Options

Exit

✓ You see the Share window.

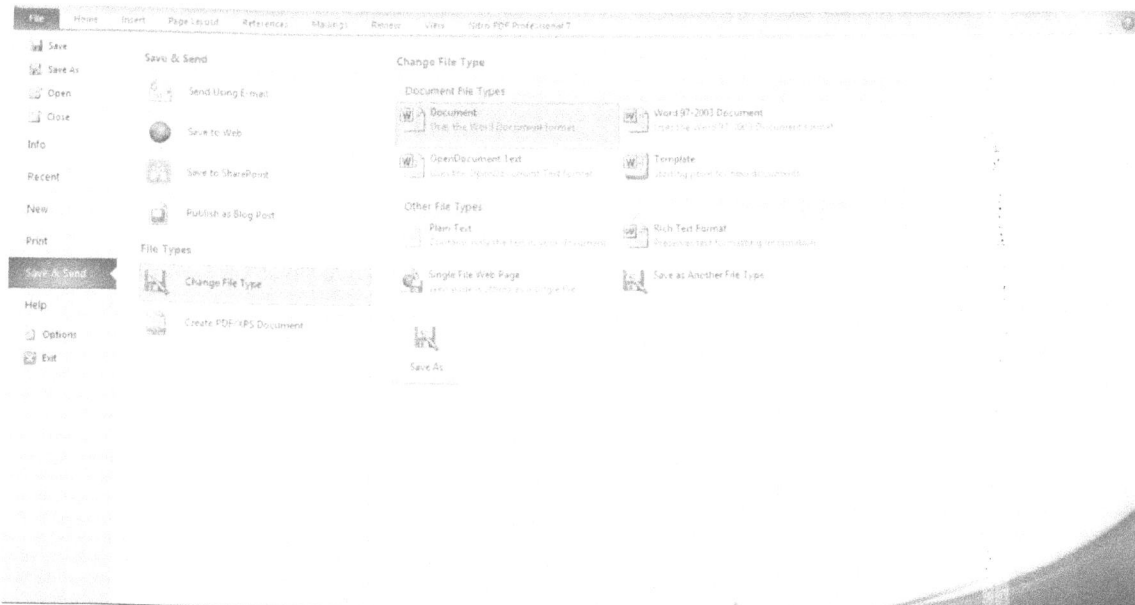

✓ Under File Types, choose Change File Type and then choose 97–2003 option for saving files. The Save As dialog box opens.

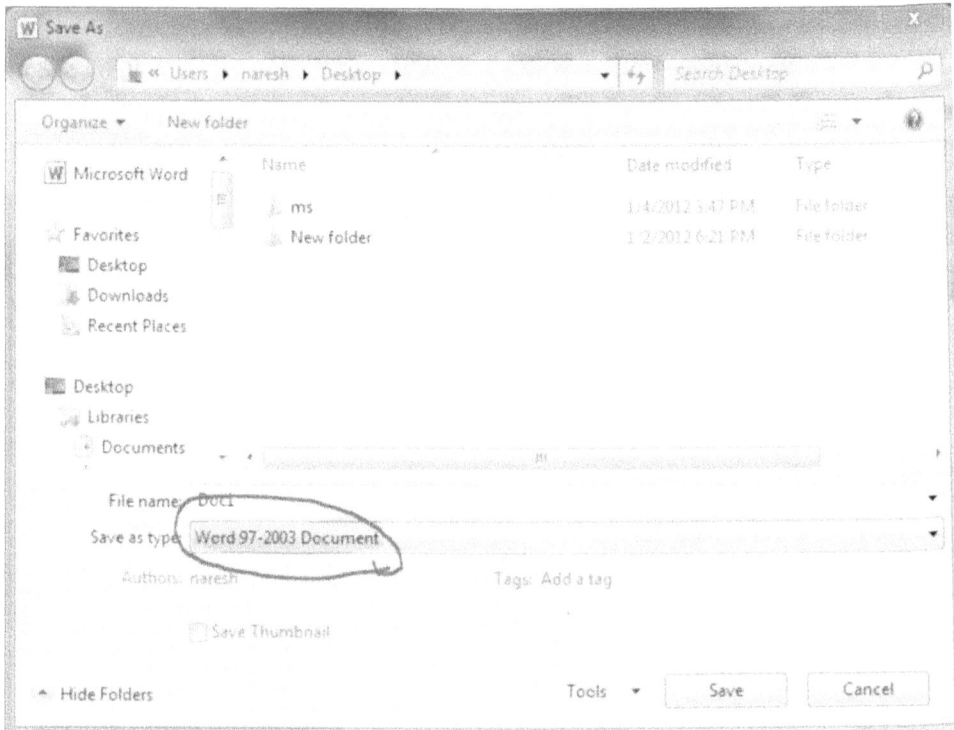

✓ Enter a new name for the file, if necessary.

✓ Click the Save button.

Saving Auto Recovery information

To insure against data loss due to computer and power failures, Office saves files on its own every ten minutes. These files are saved in an Auto Recovery file. You can try to recover some of the work you lost by getting it from the Auto Recovery file.

Convert Earlier Version of word to 2010

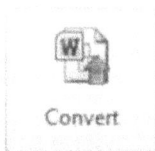

Compatibility Mode
Some new features are disabled to prevent problems when working with previous versions of Office. Converting this file will enable these features, but may result in layout changes.

Convert

Go to File → Convert→ Click "Okay"

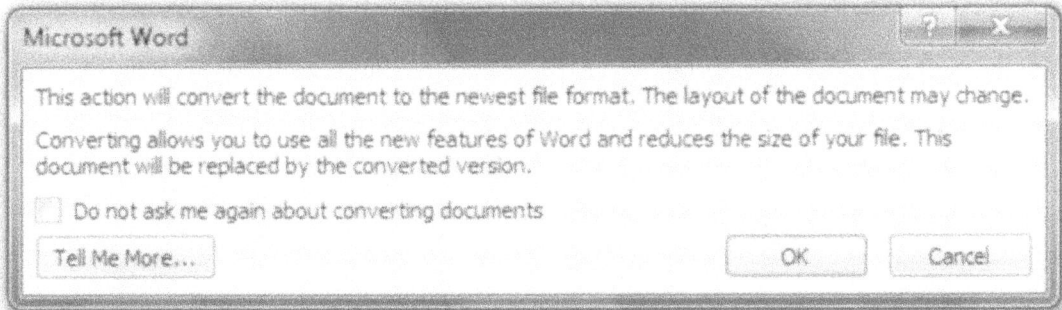

Microsoft Word

This action will convert the document to the newest file format. The layout of the document may change.

Converting allows you to use all the new features of Word and reduces the size of your file. This document will be replaced by the converted version.

☐ Do not ask me again about converting documents

Tell Me More...   OK   Cancel

The Save As and Open Dialog Boxes

The Open dialog box and Save As dialog box offer a bunch of different ways to locate a file you want to open or locate the folder where you want to save a file.

Searching for files in a folder: Use the Search box to search for subfolders and files in the folder you is currently viewing. After you type the first few letters of a file name or subfolder, you see only the names of items that start with the letters you typed. To see all the files and subfolders again, click the Close button (the X) in the Search box.

Changing views: Display folder contents differently by choosing a view on the Views drop-down list (in Windows 7, look for the View arrow in the upper-right corner of the dialog box). In Details view, you see how large files are and when they were last edited.

Creating a new folder: Click the New Folder button to create a new subfolder for storing files. Select the folder that your new folder will be subordinate to and click the New Folder button. Then type a name forthe saved file.

Navigate to different folders: Click the Folders bar (in the lower-left corner of the dialog box) to open the Navigation pane and look for folders or presentations on a different drive, network location, or folder on your computer.

Opening a file

✓ On the File tab, choose Open (or press Ctrl+O).

✓ Locate and select the file you want to open.

✓ Click the Open button.

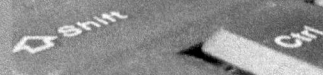

✓ Your file opens. You can also double-click a filename to open a file.

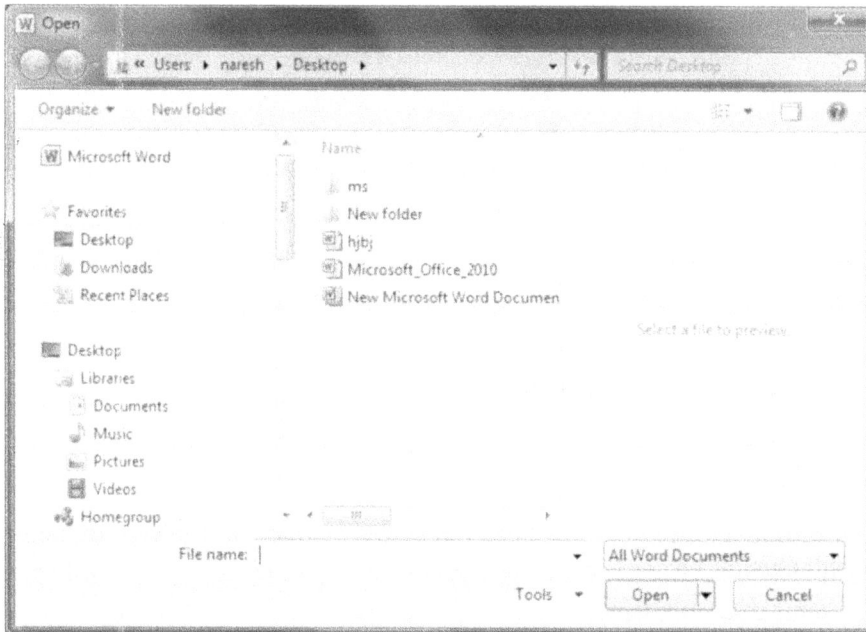

✓ If you have recently accessed the file you can use recent button in file tab.

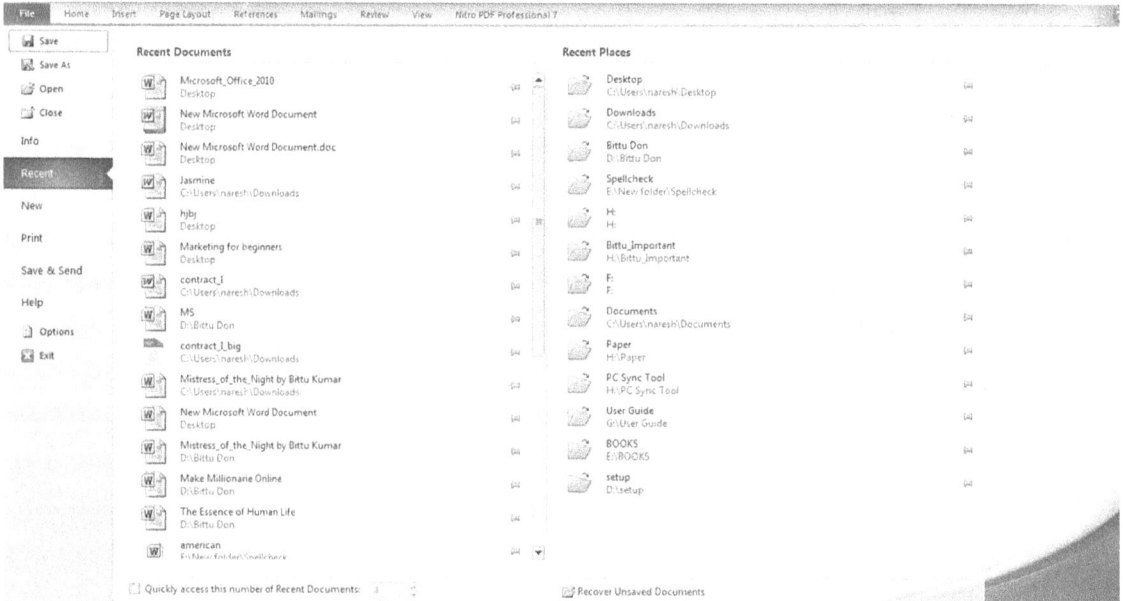

File Properties

Properties are a means of describing a file. If you manage more files, you owe it to yourself to record properties. You can use them later to identify files.

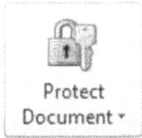

Permissions

Anyone can open, copy, and change any part of this document.

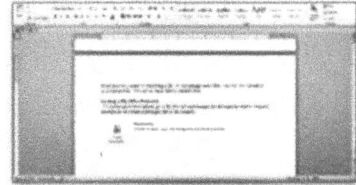

Protect Document ▾

Locking a File with a Password

Properties ▾

Size	1.28MB
Pages	20
Words	2185
Total Editing Time	155 Minutes
Title	Add a title
Tags	Add a tag
Comments	Add comments

To read property descriptions, go to the File tab and examine the Information window. Property descriptions are found on the right side of the window.

Follow these steps to clamp a password on a file, such that others need apassword to open and perhaps also edit it:

Related Dates

Last Modified	Today, 8:53 AM
Created	Yesterday, 9:25 PM
Last Printed	Never

✓ Go to the File tab.

✓ In the Information window, click the Protect Document (or Workbook) button, and choose Encrypt with Password on the drop-down list.

✓ Enter a password in the Password text box and click OK.

Others will need the password you enter to open the file. They have to enter the password.Passwords are case-sensitive. In other words, you have to enter the correct combination of upper- and lowercase letters to successfully enter the

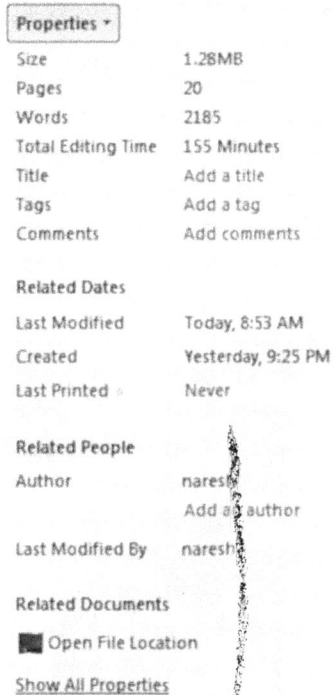

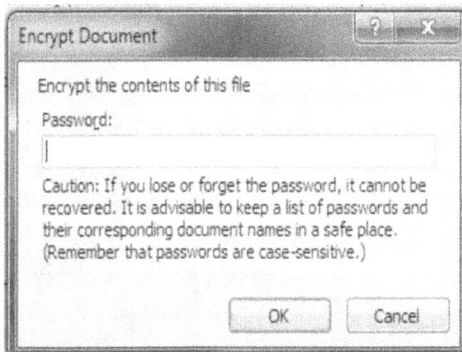

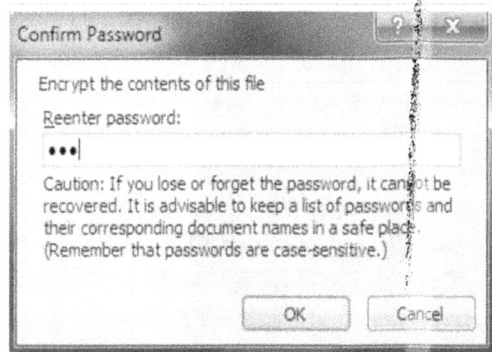

Related People

Author	naresh
	Add an author
Last Modified By	naresh

Related Documents

Open File Location

Show All Properties

Encrypt Document   ? X

Encrypt the contents of this file

Password:

| |

Caution: If you lose or forget the password, it cannot be recovered. It is advisable to keep a list of passwords and their corresponding document names in a safe place. (Remember that passwords are case-sensitive.)

OK   Cancel

Confirm Password   ? X

Encrypt the contents of this file

Reenter password:

| ••• |

Caution: If you lose or forget the password, it cannot be recovered. It is advisable to keep a list of passwords and their corresponding document names in a safe place. (Remember that passwords are case-sensitive.)

OK   Cancel

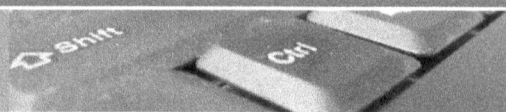

password. If the password is Apple (with an uppercase A), mentoring apple (with a lowercase a) is deemed the wrong passwordand doesn't open the file.

✓ In the Confirm Password dialog box, enter the password again.

✓ Click OK.

The Information window informs you that a password is required to open the file.

Removing Password

Follow these steps to remove a password from a file:

✓ Open the file that needs its password removed.

✓ Go to the File tab and in the Information window, click the Protect Document button, and choose Encrypt with Password.

✓ Delete the password and click OK.

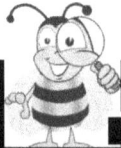

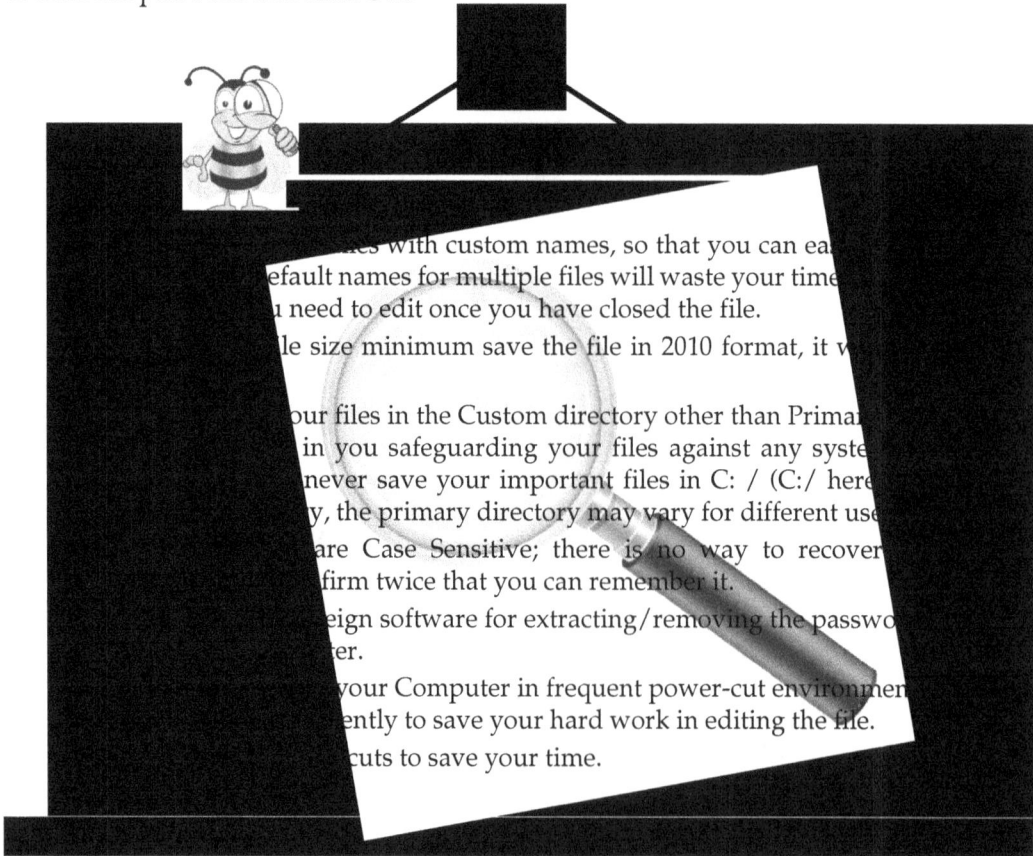

es with custom names, so that you can ea
efault names for multiple files will waste your time
need to edit once you have closed the file.
le size minimum save the file in 2010 format, it v

ur files in the Custom directory other than Prima
in you safeguarding your files against any syste
never save your important files in C: / (C:/ here
y, the primary directory may vary for different use
are Case Sensitive; there is no way to recover
firm twice that you can remember it.
eign software for extracting/removing the passwo
er.
our Computer in frequent power-cut environmen
ently to save your hard work in editing the file.
cuts to save your time.

names for saving your file, for example
ndence day, your system will give your docume
Microsoft word Document X.docx (X~ some nu
as "Independence day.docx" to remember the fil
fter quitting.

e your file at insecure places (Web directory, etc.)
ss it.

that you have an updated Anti-Malware prote
n.

the documents with your Anti-Malware softwar
probably the Files downloaded from Internet
ware, Trojan horses & some other harmful progr

ny document having other extensions than di
corrupt the file. (For example if you open pd
this will corrupt its contents.)

Formatting Text

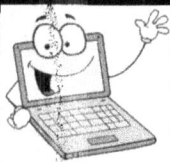

this chapter you will learn

- Ways to select different elements of the file or document
- Formatting font styles and other Elements
- Changing the size, colour, opacity of the elements in the file or document
- Using Symbols & formulae in the file or document
- Finding and replacing data in the file or document
- Creating Links to files & websites

Selecting text

Before you can perform any activity to any text you have to select it.

To Select	Do This
A word	Double-click the word.
A few words	Drag over the words.
A paragraph	Triple-click inside the paragraph
A block of text	Click the start of the text, hold down the Shift key, and click the end of the text. In Word you can also click the start of the text, press F8, and click at the end of the text.
All text	Press Ctrl+A.

Moving and Copying text

✓ **Dragging and Dropping:** Move the mouse over the text and then click and drag the text to a new location. Drag means to hold down the mouse button while you move the pointer on-screen. If you want to copy rather than move the text, hold down the Ctrl key while you drag.

✓ **Dragging and Dropping with the right mouse button**: Drag the text while holding down the right, not the left, mouse button. After you release the right mouse button, a shortcut menu appears with Move Here and Copy Here options. Choose an option to move or copy the text.

✓ **Using the Clipboard**: Move or copy the text to the Clipboard by clicking the Cut or Copy button, pressing Ctrl+X or Ctrl+C, or right-clicking and choosing Cut or Copy on the shortcut menu. The text is moved or copied to an electronic holding tank called the Clipboard. Paste the text by clicking the Paste button, pressing Ctrl+V, or right-clicking and choosing Paste. You can find the Paste, Cut, and Copy buttons on the Hometab.

Deleting text

To delete a bunch of text, select the text you want to delete and press the Delete key.

Changing the Look of Text

What text looks like is determined by its font, the size of the letters, the colour of the letters, and whether text effects or font styles such as italic or boldface are in the text. The text's appearance really matters in Word, PowerPoint, and Publisher because files you create in those programs are meant to be read by all and sundry. Even in Excel, Access, and Outlook messages, font choices matter because the choices you make determine whether your work is easy to read and understand.

A font is a collection of letters, numbers, and symbols in a particular typeface, including all italic and boldface variations of the letters, numbers, and symbols.

Choosing fonts for text

✓ **Mini-toolbar:** Move the pointer over the selected text. You see the mini toolbar. Move the pointer over this toolbar and choose a font in the Font drop-down list.

✓ **Shortcut menu:** Right-click the selected text and choose a new font on the shortcut menu.

✓ **Font drop-down list:** On the Home tab, open the Font drop-down list and choose a font.

✓ **Font dialog box:** On the Home tab, click the Font group button. You see the Font dialog box. select a font and click OK.

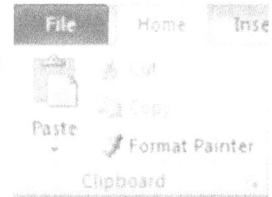

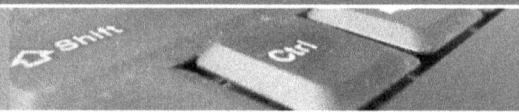

Changing the font size of text

✓ Font size is measured in points; a point is 1/72 of an inch.

✓ **Mini-toolbar:** Move the pointer over the text, and when you see the mini toolbar, move the pointer over the toolbar and choose a font size on the Font.

✓ **Shortcut menu:** Right-click the text and choose a new font size on the shortcut menu.

✓ **Font Size drop-down list:** On the Home tab, open the Font Size dropdown list and choose a font. You can live-preview font sizes this way.

✓ **Font dialog box:** On the Home tab, click the Font group button, and in the Font dialog box, choose a font size and click OK.

✓ **Increase Font Size and Decrease Font Size buttons:** Click these buttons (or press Ctrl+] or Ctrl+[) to increase or decrease the point size by the next interval on the Font Size drop-down list. A̅ A̅

Applying font styles to text

❑ **Regular:** This style is just Office's way of denoting an absence of any font style.

❑ **Italic:** You can also italicize titles to make them a little more elegant. (Ctrl+I) *I*

❑ **Bold:** Bold text calls attention to itself. (Ctrl+B) **B**

❑ **Underline:** Underlined text also calls attention to itself, but use underlining sparingly. Later in this chapter, "Underlining text" discusses all the ways to underline text. U̲ ˅

❑ **Strikethrough and double strikethrough:** By convention, strikethrough is used to show where passages are struck from a contract or other important document. a̶b̶c̶

❑ **Subscript:** A subscripted letter is lowered in the text. In the chemical formula below, the 2 is lowered to show that two atoms of hydrogen are needed along with one atom of oxygen to form a molecule of water: H_2O. (Press Ctrl+=.) $\mathbf{x}_2$

❑ **Superscript:** A superscripted letter or number is one that is raised in the text. Superscript is used in mathematical and scientific formulas, in ordinal numbers (1st, 2nd , 3rd), and to mark footnotes. In the theory of relativity, the 2 is superscripted: $E = mc^2$. (Press Ctrl+Shift+plus sign.) $\mathbf{x}^2$

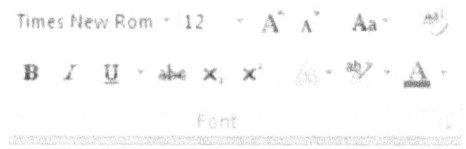

Changing the colour of text

✓ On the mini-toolbar, open the drop-down list on the Font Colour button and choose a colour.

A ˅

✓ Right-click, open the drop-down list on the Font Colour button, and choose a colour on the shortcut menu.

✓ On the Home tab, open the drop-down list on the Font Colour button and choose a colour.

✓ On the Home tab, click the Font group button to open the Font dialog box, open the Font Colour drop-down list, and choose a colour. The Font Colour drop-down list offers theme colours and standard colours. You are well advised to choose a theme colour. These colours are deemed theme colours because they jive with the theme you choose for your file.

Changing Case

To change case in Word and PowerPoint, all you have to do is select the text, go to the Home tab, click the Change Case button, and choose an option on the drop-down list:

❑ **Sentence case:** Renders the letters in sentence case.

❑ **lowercase:** Makes all the letters lowercase.

❑ **UPPERCASE:** Renders all the letters as capital letters.

❑ **Capitalize Each Word:** Capitalizes the first letter of each word. If you choose this option for a title or heading, go into the title and lower case the first letter of articles (the, a, an), coordinate conjunctions (and, or, for, nor), and prepositions unless they're the first or last word in the title.

❑ **TOGGLE CASE:** Choose this option if you accidentally enter letters with the Caps Lock key pressed.

Entering Symbols and Foreign Characters

✓ On the Insert tab, click the Symbol button. (You may have to click the Symbols button first, depending on the size of your screen)

✓ If you're looking to insert a symbol, not a foreign character, choose Webdings or Wingdings 1, 2, or 3 in the Font drop-down list.

✓ Webdings and Wingdings fonts offer all kinds of weird and wacky symbols.

✓ Select a symbol or foreign character.

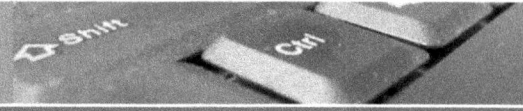

✓ Click the Insert button to enter the symbol and then click Close to close the dialog box.

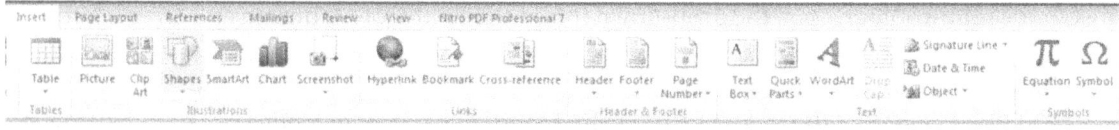

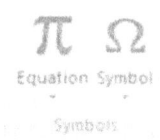

Finding and Replacing Text

✓ Press Ctrl+F or go to the Home tab and click the Find button. (In Excel, click the Find & Select button and choose Find on the dropdown list.)

✓ Enter the word or phrase in the Find What or Search Documenttext box.

After you enter the word or phrase in Word, the Navigation pane lists each instance of the term you're looking for and the term is highlighted in your document wherever it is found. You can click an instance of the search term in the Navigation pane to scroll to a location in your document where the search term is located. You can also remove the word using replace.

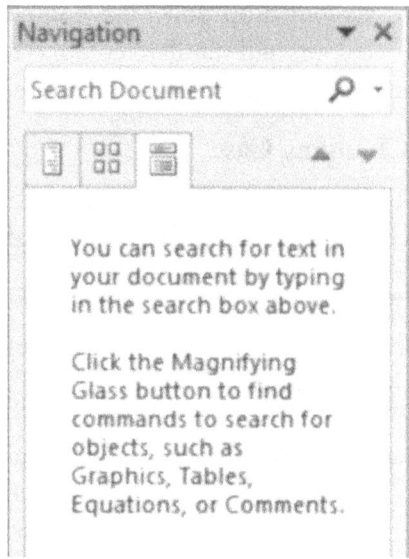

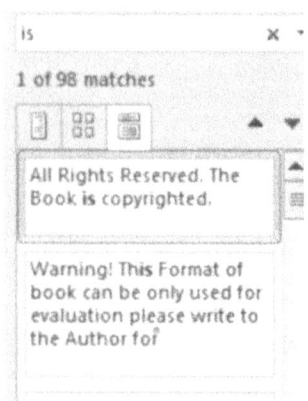

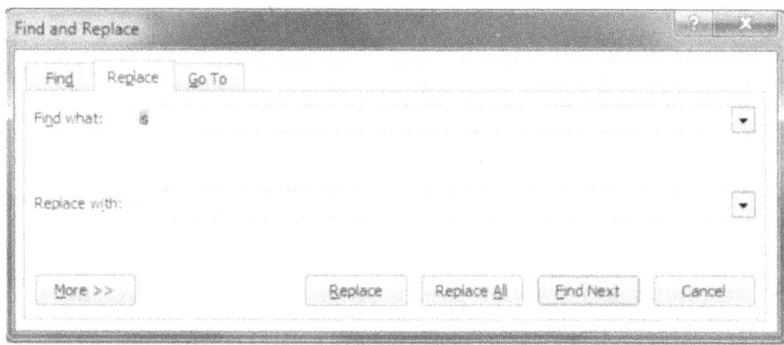

Finding and Replacing text

Creating Hyperlinks

A hyperlink is an electronic shortcut from one place to another. Clicking hyperlinks on the Internet takes you to different web pages or different places on the same web page. In the Office programs, you can use hyperlinks to connect readers to your favourite web pages or to a different page, slide, or file.

Hyperlink

Select the text or object that will form the hyperlink.

For example, select a line of text or phrase if you want viewers to be able to click it to go to a web page.

✓ On the Insert tab, click the Hyperlink button (or press Ctrl+K). Depending on the size of your screen, you may have to click the Links button before you can get to the Hyperlink button. You can also open this dialog box by right-clicking an object or text and choosing Hyperlink on the shortcut menu

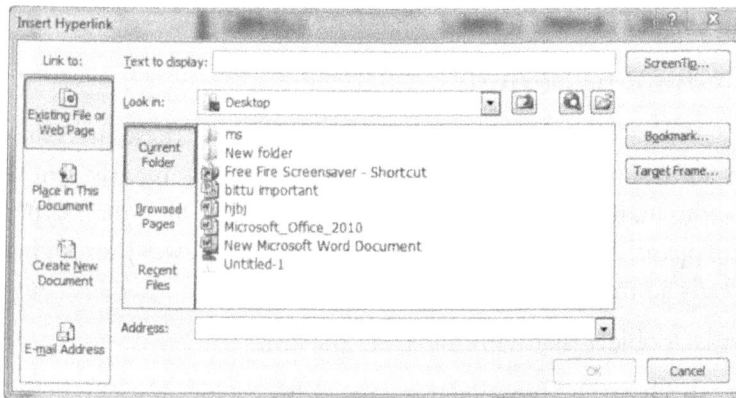

Creating Hyperlink

✓ **Click Browse the Web button:** Your web browser opens after you click this button. Go to the web page you want to link to and return to your program. The web page's address appears in the Address text box.

✓ **Click Browsed Pages:** The dialog box lists web pages you recently visited after you click this button, Type (or copy) a web page address into the Address text box: Enter the address of the web page. You can right-click the text box and choose Paste to copy a web page address into the text box.

✓ Click the ScreenTip button, enter a ScreenTip in the Set HyperlinkScreenTip dialog box, and click OK.

✓ Click OK in the Insert Hyperlink dialog box.

Creating a hyperlink to another place in your file

Follow these steps to create a hyperlink to another place in your file:

✓ Select the text or object that will form the hyperlink.

✓ On the Insert tab, click the Hyperlink button (or press Ctrl+K). You see the Insert Hyperlink dialog box. Another way to open this dialog box is to right-click and choose Hyperlink in the shortcut menu.

✓ Under Link To, select Place in This Document. What you see in the dialog box depends on which program you're working in.

✓ Select the target of the hyperlink. Click the ScreenTip button.

✓ You see the Set Hyperlink ScreenTip dialog box.

✓ Enter a ScreenTip and click OK. When viewers move their pointers over the link, they see the words you enter. Enter a description of where the hyperlink takes you.

Creating an e-mail hyperlink

✓ An e-mail hyperlink is one that opens an e-mail program. These links are sometimes found on web pages so that anyone visiting a web page can conveniently send an e-mail message to the person who manages the web page. When you click an e-mail hyperlink, your default e-mail program opens. And If the person who set up the link was thorough about it, the e-mail message is already addressed and given a subject line.

✓ Select the words or object that will constitute the link.

✓ On the Insert tab, click the Hyperlink button (or press Ctrl+K). The Insert Hyperlink dialog box appears.

✓ Under Link To, click E-Mail Address. Text boxes appear for entering an e-mail address and a subject message.

✓ Enter your e-mail address and a subject for the messages that others will send you. Office inserts the word mail to: before your e-mail address as you enter it.

✓ Click OK.

Repairing and removing hyperlinks

✓ **Repairing a link:** Select a target in your file or a web page and click OK.

✓ **Removing a link:** Click the Remove Link button. You can also remove a hyperlink by right-clicking the link and choosing Remove.

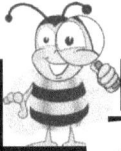

ng skills at your best
king, double check th
king make sure that
ons

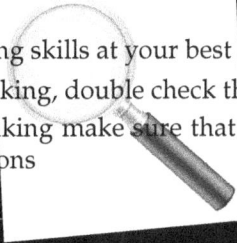

4th Chapter

Get more from Office

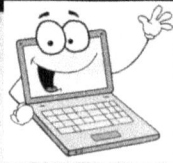

this chapter you will learn

- Tracking changes to a document or file
- Accessibility options in Microsoft office 2010
- Using language Tools

Undoing and Repeating Commands

Undo allows you to reverse actions you regret doing, and the Repeat repeats a previous action without you have to choose the same commands all over again. All is not lost if you make a big blunder because Office has a marvelous little tool called the Undo command. This command "Remembers" your previous editorial and formatting changes. As long as you catch your error in time, you can undo your mistake.

✓ Click the Undo button on the Quick Access toolbar (or press Ctrl+Z) to undo your most recent change. If you made your error and went on to do something else before you caught it, open the drop-down list on the Undo button.

✓ Click Redo to redo the change.

Zooming

You can find these controls in the lower-right corner of the window and on the View tab

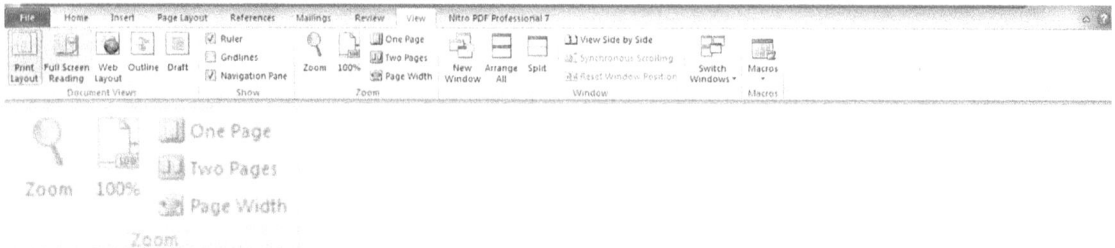

- **Zoom dialog box:** Click the Zoom button on the View tab or the Zoom box (the % listing) to display the Zoom dialog box; you can select an option button or enter a Percent measurement.

- **Zoom button:** Click the Zoom In or Zoom Out button on the Zoom slider to zoom in or out in 10-percent increments.

- **Zoom slider:** Drag the Zoom slider left to shrink or right to enlarge what is on your screen.

- **Mouse wheel:** If your mouse has a wheel, you can hold down the Ctrl key and spin the wheel to quickly zoom in or out.

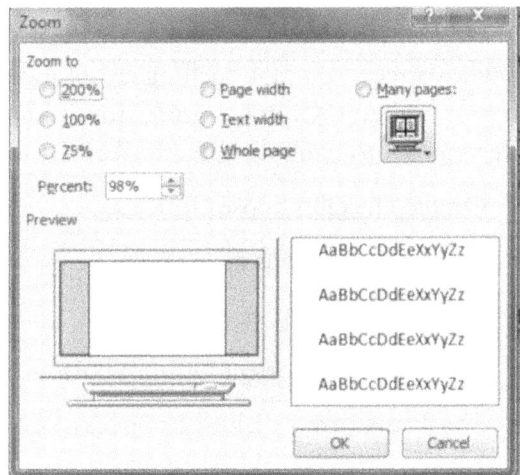

Zooming text

Viewing a File through more than One Window

- **New Window:** Opens another window on your file, so that you can view two places simultaneously in the same file. To go back and forth between windows, click a taskbar button or click the Switch Windows button and choose a window name on the drop-down list. Click window's Close button when you're finished looking at it.

Viewing a file through more than one window

- **Arrange All:** Arranges open windows side by side on-screen.

- **Switch Windows:** Opens a drop-down list with open windows so that you can travel between windows.

- **View Side by Side:** Displays files side by side so that you can compare and contrast them.

- **Synchronous Scrolling:** Permits you to scroll two files at the same rate so that you can proofread one against the other. To use this command, start by clicking the View Side by Side button. After you click the Synchronous Scrolling button, click the Reset Window Position button so both files are displayed at the same size on-screen.

- **Reset Window Position:** Makes files being shown side by side the same size on-screen to make them easier to compare.

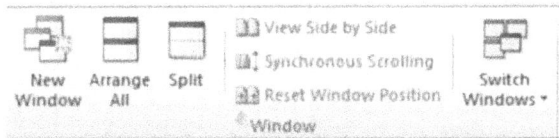

Opening AutoCorrect dialog box

Office corrects common spelling errors and turns punctuation mark combinations into symbols as part of its AutoCorrect feature. To see which typos are corrected and which punctuation marks are turned into symbols, open the AutoCorrect dialog box by following these steps:

✓ On the File tab, choose Options.

✓ You see the Options dialog box.

✓ Go to the Proofing category.

✓ Click the AutoCorrect Options button.

✓ The AutoCorrect dialog box opens.

✓ Click the AutoCorrect tab.

✓ AutoCorrect tab lists words that are corrected automatically. Scroll down the Replace list and have a look around. Go ahead and make yourself at home.

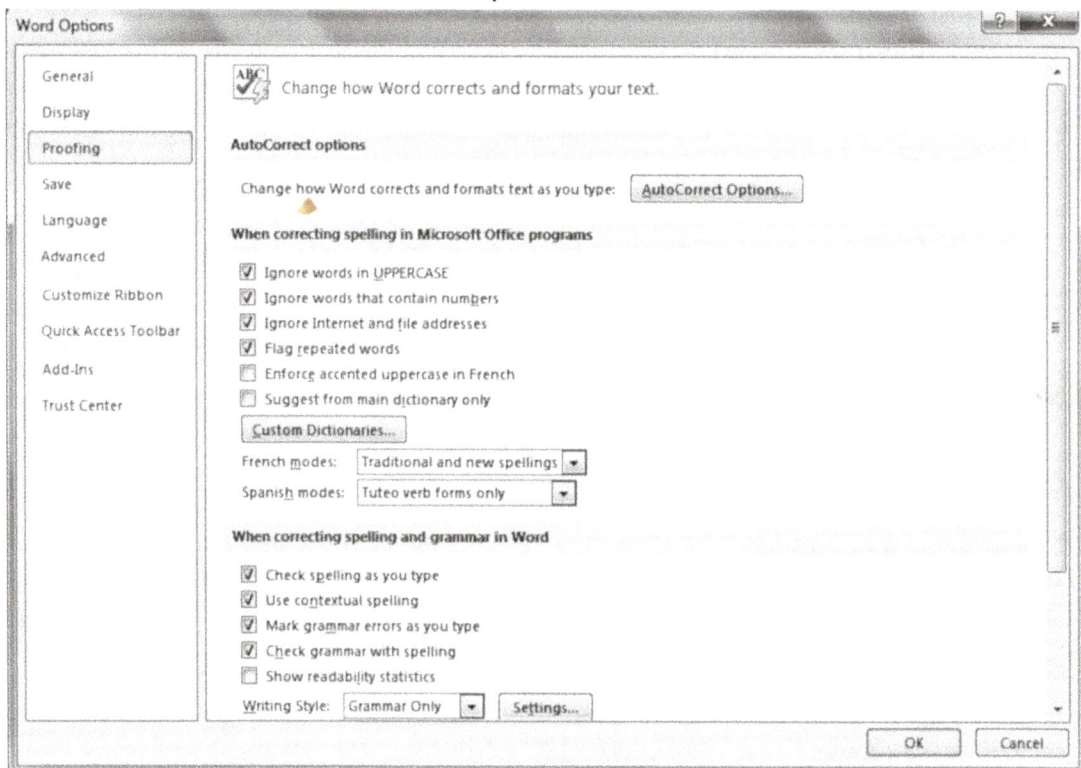

Auto correct dialog box

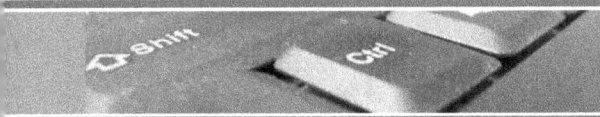

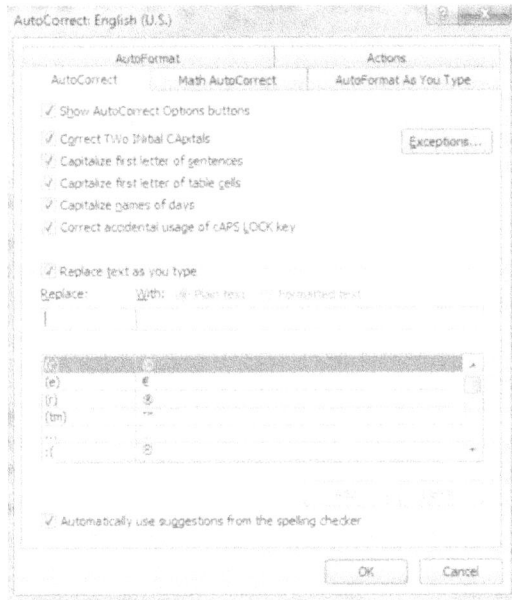

Checking for Grammatical Errors in Word

You can do your best to repair grammatical errors in Word documents by getting the assistance of the grammar checker. The grammar checker identifies grammatical errors, explains what the errors are, and gives you the opportunity to correct the errors. Sentences in which grammatical errors appear are underlined in blue in your document. Meanwhile, the grammatical errors themselves appear in bright blue in the box at the top of the Spelling and Grammar dialog box (alongwith spelling errors, which are red). When Word encounters an error, take one of these actions to correct it:

✓ Select a correction in the Suggestions box and click the Change button.

✓ Delete the grammatical error or rephrase the sentence in the top of the dialog box, enter a correction, and click the Change button.

✓ Click outside the Spelling and Grammar dialog box, correct the grammatical error in your document, and then click the Resume button (you find it where the Ignore Once button used to be).

Click one of the Ignore buttons to let what Word thinks is a grammatical error stand.

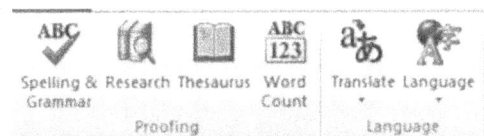

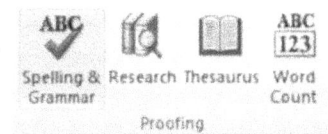

Researching a Topic inside an Office Program

Thanks to the Research task pane, your desk needn't be as crowded as before. The Research task pane offers dictionaries, foreign language dictionaries, a thesaurus, language translators, and encyclopedias, as well as Internet searching, all available from inside the Office programs.

Finding the Right Word with the Thesaurus

To search for a good synonym, click the word in question and open the thesaurus on the Research task pane with one of these techniques:

✓ Press Shift+F7.

✓ Right-click the word and choose Synonym → Thesaurus.

✓ Go to the Review tab and click the Thesaurus button.

The Research task pane opens. It offers a list of synonyms and sometimes includes an antonym or two at the bottom. Now you're getting somewhere:

❑ **Choosing a synonym:** Move the pointer over the synonym you want, open its drop-down list, and choose Insert.

❑ **Finding a synonym for a synonym:** If a synonym intrigues you, click it. The task pane displays a new list of synonyms.

❑ **Searching for antonyms:** If you can't think of the right word, type its antonym in the Search For box and then look for an "antonym of an antonym" in the Research task pane.

❑ **Revisit a word list:** Click the Back button as many times as necessary. If you go back too far, you can always click its companion Forward button.

Telling Office which languages you will use

Follow these steps to inform Word, PowerPoint, Publisher, and Outlook that you will use a language or languages besides English in your files:

✓ On the Review tab, click the Language button and choose Language Preferences. The Options dialog box opens to the Language category.

Language

✓ Open the Add Additional Editing Languages drop-down list, select a language, and click the Add button to make that language a part of your presentations, documents, and messages.

✓ Click OK.

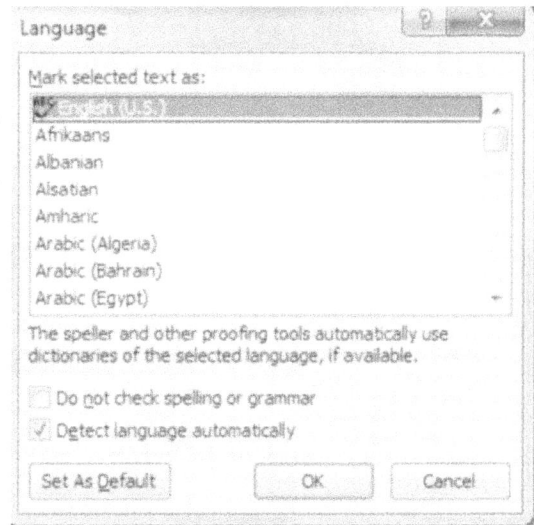

Marking text as foreign language text

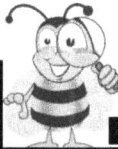

The next step is to tell Office where in your file you're using a foreign language. After you mark the text as foreign language text, Office can spellcheck it with the proper dictionaries. Follow these steps to mark text so that Office knows in which language it was written:

✓ Select the text that you wrote in a foreign language.

✓ Go to the Review tab.

✓ Click the Language button and choose Set Proofing Language on the drop-down list.

✓ Select a language and click OK.

Marking text as foreign language text

ce provides limited supp
nts and custom dictionaries
egional keyboard thorough
rammar checker for best re
r saving your time

Tables

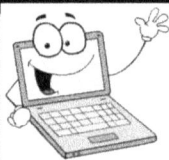

this chapter you will learn

- Using table tools
- Utilising other Table Resources

Before starting the Course you need to know the following terms:

❏ **Cell:** The box that is formed where a row and column intersect. Each cell holds one data item.

❏ **Header row:** The name of the labels along the top row that explain what is in the columns below.

❏ **Row labels:** The labels in the first column that describe what is in each row.

❏ **Borders:** The lines in the table that define where the rows and columns are.

❏ **Gridlines:** The gray lines that show where the columns and rows are.

Unless you've drawn borders around all the cells in a table, you can't tell where rows and columns begin and end without gridlines. To display or hide the gridlines, go to the (Table Tools) Layout tab and click the View Gridlines button.

Creating a Table

❏ **Drag on the Table menu:** On the Insert tab, click the Table button, point in the drop-down list to the number of columns and rows you want, click, and let go of the mouse button.

Row labels		Header row		
	Qtr 1	Qtr 2	Qtr 3	Qtr 4
East	4	8	5	6
West	3	4	4	9
North	3	8	9	6
South	8	7	7	9

Borders   Gridlines   Cells

❑ **Use the Insert Table dialog box:** On the Insert tab, click the Table button and choose Insert Table on the drop-down list. The Insert Table dialog box appears. Enter the number of columns and rows you want and click OK. In PowerPoint, you can also open the Insert Table dialog box by clicking the Table icon in a content placeholder frame.

❑ **Draw a table (Word and PowerPoint):** On the Insert tab, click the Table button and then choose Draw Table on the drop-down list. The pointer changes into a pencil. Use the pencil to draw table borders, rows, and columns. If you make a mistake, click the Eraser button on the (Table Tools) Design tab and drag it over the parts of the table you regret drawing (you may have to click the Draw Borders button first). When you finish drawing the table, press Esc. You can click the Pen Colour button and choose a colour on the drop-down list to draw your table in your favourite colour.

❑ **Create a quick table (Word):** On the Insert tab, click the Table button and choose Quick Tables on the drop-down list. Then choose a readymade table on the submenu. You have to replace the sample data in the quick table with your own data.

❑ **Convert text in a list into a table (Word):** Press Tab or enter a comma in each list item where you want the columns in the table to be. Select the text you'll convert to a table, click the Table button on the Insert tab, and choose Convert Text to Table. Under Separate Text At in the Convert Text to Table dialog box, choose Tabs or Commas to tell Word how the columns are separated. Then click OK.

Entering Text and Numbers

After you create the table, you can start entering text and numbers. All you have to do is click in a cell and start typing. Select your table and take advantage of these methods to make the onerous task of entering table data a little easier:

❑ **Quickly changing a table's size:** Drag the bottom or side of a table to change its overall size. In Word, you can also go to the (Table Tools) Layout tab, click the AutoFit button, and choose AutoFit Window to make the table stretch from margin to margin.

❑ **Moving a table:** In Word, switch to Print Layout view and drag the table selector (the square in the upper-left corner of the table). In PowerPoint and Publisher, move the pointer over the table's perimeter, and when you see the four-headed arrow, click and drag.

❑ **Choosing your preferred font and font size:** Entering table data is easier when you're working in a font and font size you like. Select the table, visit the Home tab, and choose a font and font size there. In Word and PowerPoint, you can select a table by going to the (Table Tools) Layout tab, clicking the Select button, and choosing Select Table on the drop-down list.

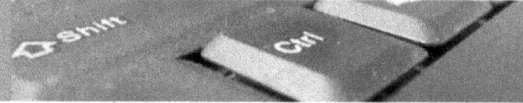

❏ Quickly inserting a new row: Click in the last column of the last row in your table and press the Tab key to quickly insert a new row at the bottom of the table.

Selecting different parts of a Table

❏ **Selecting cells:** To select a cell, click it. You can select several adjacent cells by dragging the pointer over them.

❏ **Selecting rows:** Move the pointer to the left of the row and click when you see the right-pointing arrow; click and drag to select several rows. You can also go to the (Table Tools) Layout tab, click inside the row you want to select, click the Select button, and choose Select Row on the drop-down list. To select more than one row at a time, select cells in the rows before choosing the Select Row command.

❏ **Selecting columns:** Move the pointer above the column and click when you see the down-pointing arrow; click and drag to select several columns. You can also start from the (Table Tools) Layout tab, click in the column you want to select, click the Select button, and choose Select Column in the drop-down list. To select several columns, select cells in the columns before choosing the Select Column command.

❏ **Selecting a table:** On the (Table Tools) Layout tab, click the Select button, and choose Select Table on the drop-down list. In PowerPoint, you can also right-click a table and choose Select Table on the shortcut menu.

Merging and Splitting Cells

Merge cells to break down the barriers between cells and join them into one cell; split cells to divide a single cell into several cells (or severalcells into several more cells).

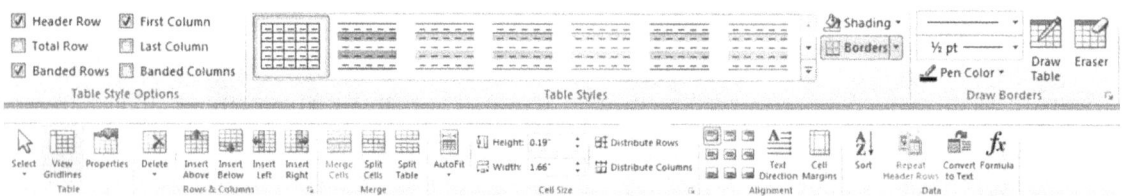

❏ Select the cells you want to merge or split, go to the (Table Tools) Layout tab, and follow these instructions to merge or split cells:

   ✓ **Merging cells:** Click the Merge Cells button (in Word and PowerPoint, you can also right-click and choose Merge Cells).

   ✓ **Splitting cells:** Click the Split Cells button (in Word and PowerPoint, you can also right-click and choose Split Cells). In the Split Cells dialog box, declare how many columns and rows you want to split the cell into and then click OK. In Publisher, you can only split cells that were previously merged.

Laying Out your Table

❑ **Column or row:** Move the pointer onto a gridline or border, and when the pointer changes into a double-headed arrow, start dragging. Tug and pull, tug and pull until the column or row is the right size. In Word and PowerPoint, you can also go to the (Table Tools) Layout tab and enter measurements in the Height and Width text boxes to change the width of a column or the height of a row. The measurements affect entire columns or rows, not individual cells.

❑ **A table:** Select your table and use one of these techniques to change its size in Word and PowerPoint:

❑ **Dragging:** Drag the top, bottom, or side of the table. You can also drag the lower-right corner to change the size vertically and horizontally.

❑ **Height and Width text boxes:** On the (Table Tools) Layout tab, enter measurements in the Height and Width text boxes. In Publisher, these text boxes are found on the (Table Tools) Design tab. In PowerPoint, click the Lock Aspect Ratio check box if you want to keep the table's proportions when you change its height or width.

❑ **Table Properties dialog box (Word only):** On the (Table Tools) Layout tab, click the Cell Size group button, and on the Table tab of the Table Properties dialog box, enter a measurement in the Preferred Width text box.

Adjusting Column and Row size

Resizing columns and rows can be problematic in Word and PowerPoint. For that reason, Word and PowerPoint offer special commands on the (Table Tools) Layout tab for adjusting the width and height of rows and columns:

❑ **Making all columns the same width:** Click the Distribute Columns button to make all columns the same width. Select columns before giving this command to make only the columns you select the same width.

❑ **Making all rows the same height:** Click the Distribute Rows button to make all rows in the table the same height. Select rows before clicking the button to make only the rows you select the same height. In Word, you can also click the AutoFit button on the (Table Tools) Layout tab, and take advantage of these commands on the drop-down list for handling columns and rows.

❑ **AutoFit Contents:** Make each column wide enough to accommodate its widest entry.

- **AutoFit Window:** Stretch the table so that it fits across the page between the left and right margin.
- **Fixed Column Width:** Fix the column widths at their current settings.

Inserting and deleting columns and rows

- **Inserting columns:** Select a column or columns and click the Insert Left or Insert Right button. If you want to insert just one column, click in a column and then click the Insert Left or Insert Right button. You can also right-click, choose Insert, and choose an Insert Columns command.
- **Inserting rows:** Select a row or rows and click the Insert Above or Insert Below button. If you want to insert just one row, click in a row and click the Insert Above or Insert Below button. You can also right-click, choose Insert, and choose an Insert Rows command on the shortcut menu. To insert a row at the end of a table, move the pointer into the last cell in the last row and press the Tab key.
- **Deleting columns:** Click in the column you want to delete, click the Delete button, and choose Delete Columns on the drop-down list. Select more than one column to delete more than one. (Pressing the Delete key deletes the data in the column, not the column itself.)
- **Deleting rows:** Click in the row you want to delete, click the Delete button, and choose Delete Rows. Select more than one row to delete more than one. (Pressing the Delete key deletes the data in the row, not the row itself.)

Moving Columns and Rows

To move a column or row:

- Select the column or row you want to move. Earlier in this chapter, "Selecting Different Parts of a Table" explains how to select columns and rows.
- Right-click in the selection and choose Cut on the shortcut menu. The column or row is moved to the Clipboard.
- Insert a new column or row where you want the column or row to be. Earlier in this chapter, "Inserting and deleting columns and rows" explains how.

Move the whole column or row:

- **Column:** Click in the topmost cell in your new column and then click the Paste button or press Ctrl+V.
- **Row:** Click in the first column of the row you inserted and then click the Paste button or press Ctrl+V.

Designing a table with a table style

Click anywhere in your table and follow these steps to choose a table style:

✓ Go to the (Table Tools) Design tab.

✓ Open the Table Styles gallery and move the pointer over table style choices to "live-preview" the table. In Publisher, this gallery is called Table Formats.

✓ Select a table style. To remove a table style, open the Table Styles gallery and choose Clear (in Word) or Clear Table (in PowerPoint).

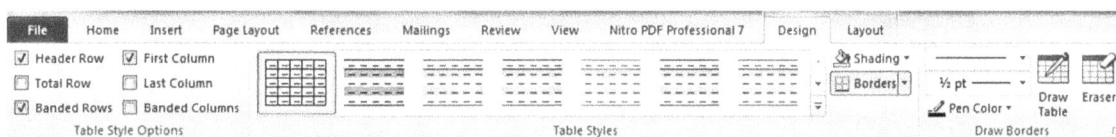

Designing borders for your table

Follow these steps to fashion a border for your table or a part of your table:

✓ Go to the (Table Tools) Design tab.

✓ Select the part of your table that needs a new border.

To select the entire table, go to the (Table Tools) Layout tab, click the Select button, and choose Select Table.

✓ Open the Line Style drop-down list (in Word) or the Pen Style drop down list (in PowerPoint) and choose a line style for the border (you may have to click the Draw Borders button first, depending on the size of your screen). Stay away from the dotted and dashed lines unless you have a good reason for choosing one. These lines can be distracting and keep others from focusing on the data presented in the table.

✓ Open the Line Weight drop-down list (in Word and Publisher) or the Pen Weight drop-down list (in PowerPoint) and choose a thickness for the border (you may have to click the Draw Borders button first).

✓ If you want your borders to be of another colour apart from black, click the Pen Colour button (Word and PowerPoint) or the Line Colour button (Publisher) and choose a colour on the drop-down list (you may have to click the Draw Borders button first).

✓ Open the drop-down list on the Borders button and choose where to place borders on the part of the table you selected in Step 2.

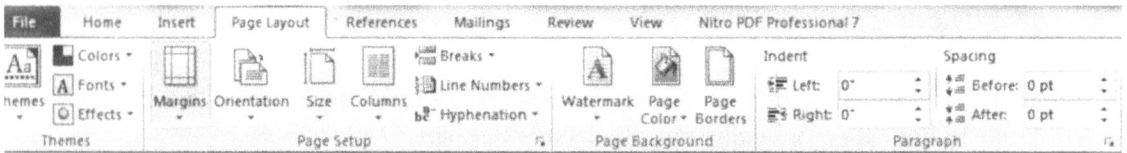

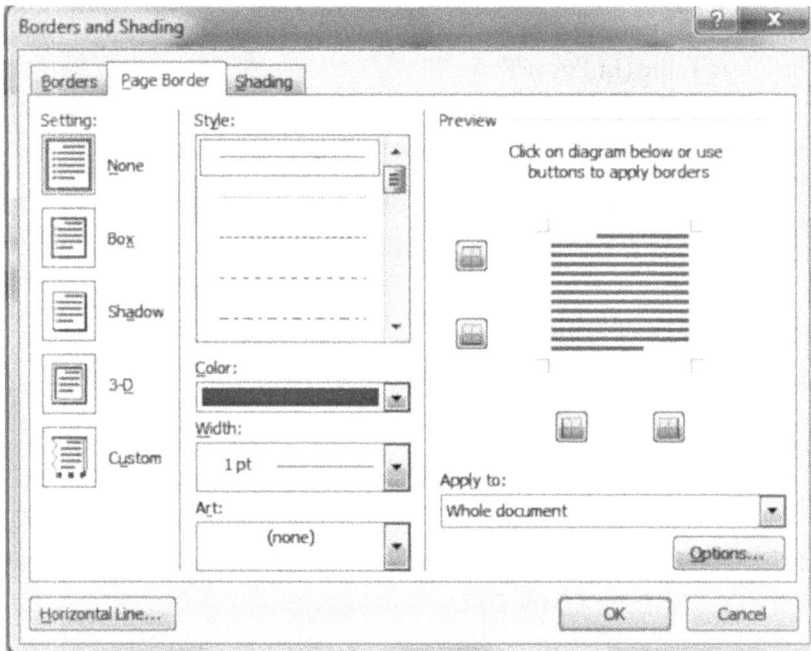

Using Math Formulas in Word Tables

You don't have to add the figures in columns and rows yourself; Word gladly does that for you. Word can perform other mathematical calculationsas well. Follow these steps to perform mathematical calculations and tell Word how to format sums and products:

✓ Put the cursor in the cell that will hold the sum or product of the cells above, below, to the right, or to the left.

✓ On the (Table Tools) Layout tab, click the Formula button.

Drawing diagonal lines on tables

Draw diagonal lines across table cells to cancel out those cells or otherwise make cells look different.

❑ **Draw Table button:** Click the Draw Table button (you may have to click the Draw Borders button first). The pointer changes into a pencil. Drag to draw the diagonal lines. Press Esc or click the Draw Table button a second time when you're finished drawing. Click the Pen Colour button and choose a colour before drawing on your table if you want the diagonal lines to be of certain colour.

❑ **Borders button:** Select the cells that need diagonal lines, open the dropdown list on the Borders button, and choose Diagonal down Border or Diagonal Up Border.

Drawing on a Table

✓ On the Insert tab, click the Shapes button and select the Oval shape on the drop-down list.

✓ On a corner of your page or slide, away from the table, drag to draw the oval.

✓ On the (Drawing Tools) Format tab, open the drop-down list on the Shape Fill button and choose No Fill.

✓ Open the drop-down list on the Shape Outline button and choose a very dark colour.

✓ Open the drop-down list on the Shape Outline button, choose Weight, and choose a thick line.

✓ Drag the oval over the data on your table that you want to highlight. If the oval is obscured by the table, go to the (Drawing Tools) Format tab, and click the Bring Forward button (click the Arrange button, if necessary,to see this button). While you're at it, consider rotating the oval a little way to make it appear as though it was drawn by hand on the table.

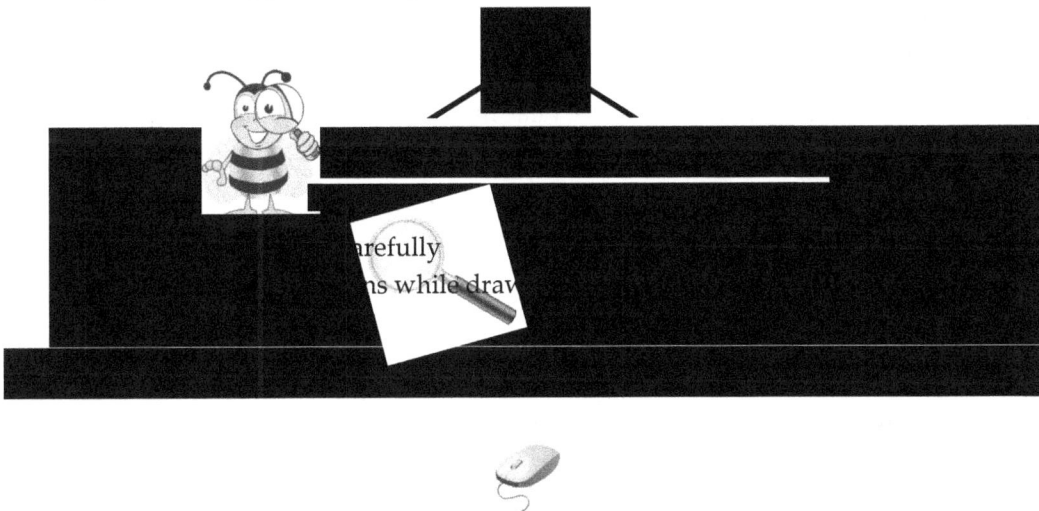

Charts

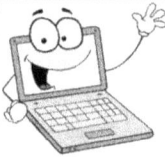

this chapter you will learn

- Using Charts
- Creating & designing charts
- Using other Graphical effects in your file

Anatomy of Charts

Before you start doing activities on charts, you need to know the following:

❑ **Plot area:** The center of the chart, apart from the legend and data labels, where the data itself is presented.

❑ **Values:** The numerical values with which the chart is plotted. The values you enter determine the size of the data markers — the bars, columns, pie slices, and so on — that portray values.

❑ **Gridlines:** Lines on the chart that indicate value measurements. Gridlines are optional in charts.

❑ **Worksheet:** Where you enter (or retrieve) the data used to plot the chart. The worksheet resembles a table. A worksheet is called a data table when it appears along with a chart.

❑ **Data series:** A group of related data points presented by category on a chart.

❑ **Categories:** The actual items that you want to compare or display in your chart.

❑ **Legend:** A text box located to the side, top, or bottom of a chart that identifies the chart's data labels.

❑ **Horizontal and vertical axes:** For plotting purposes, one side of the plot area.

❑ **Data point:** A value plotted on a chart that is represented by a column, line, bar, pie slice, dot, or other shape.

- ❑ **Data marker:** Shapes on a chart that represents data points.

- ❑ **Data label:** A label that shows the actual values used to construct the data markers.

The Basics: Creating a Chart

✓ Go to the Insert tab.

✓ If you're working in Excel, select the data you'll use to generate the chart.

✓ Select the kind of chart you want.

✓ To modify your chart, start by selecting it. Click a chart to select it. Selecting a chart makes the Chart Tools tabs appear in the upper-right corner of the window. Use these tabs — Design, Layout, and Format — to make your chart just-so. In Word, you must be in Print Layout view to see a chart.

✓ Select the (Chart Tools) Design tab when you want to change the chart's layout, alter the data with which the chart was generated, or select a different chart type.

✓ Select the (Chart Tools) Layout tab when you want to change the chart's title, labels, or gridlines. You can add or remove parts of a chart starting on the Layout tab.

✓ Select the (Chart Tools) Format tab when you want to change the appearance of your chart.

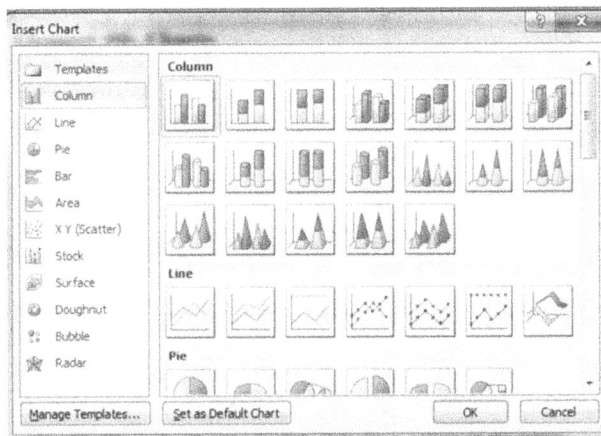

Changing chart layout

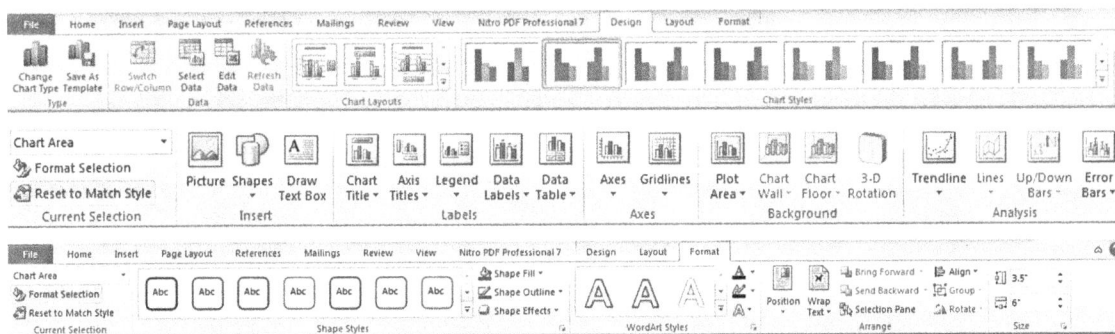

- ❑ **Design tab:** For quickly changing a chart's appearance, go to the Design tab. The ready-made gallery choices give you the opportunity to change a chart's layout and appearance in a matter of seconds. You can also choose a new chart type from the Design tab.

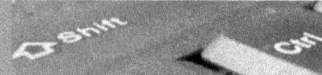

❑ **Layout tab:** For rearranging, hiding, and displaying various parts of a chart, including the legend, labels, title, gridlines, and scale, go to the Layout tab to tweak your chart and make different parts of it stand out or recede into the background.

❑ **Format tab:** For changing the colour, outline, font, and font size of various parts of a chart, including the labels, bars, and pie slices, you have to really know what you're doing and have a lot of time on your hands to change colours and fonts throughout a chart.

Changing Chart Type

✓ Click your chart to select it.

✓ On the (Chart Tools) Design tab, click the Change Chart Type button, or right-click your chart and choose Change Chart Type on the shortcut menu.

✓ Select a new chart type and click OK.

Changing Size and Shape of a Chart

To make a chart taller or wider, follow these instructions:

✓ Click the perimeter of the chart to select it and then drag a handle on the side to make it wider, or a handle on the top or bottom to make it taller.

✓ Go to the (Chart Tools) Format tab and enter measurements in the Shape Height and Shape Width boxes. You can find these boxes in the Size group (you may have to click the Size button to see them, depending on the size of your screen).

Relying on A Chart Style to change appearances

The easiest way to change the look of a chart is to choose an option in the Chart Styles gallery in the (Chart Tools) Design tab.

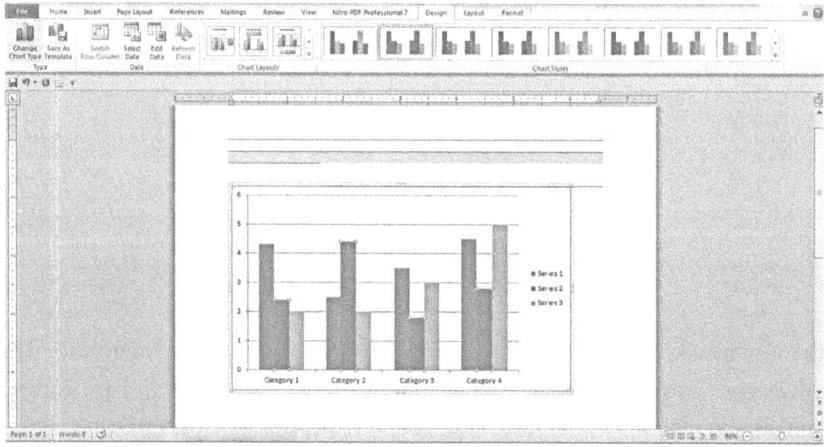

Changing a Chart elements' colour, font, or other particular

✓ Select the (Chart Tools) Format tab. The tools on the (Chart Tools) Format tab are very similar to the tools found on the (Drawing Tools) Format tab. You can find all the tools you need here to change the colour, outline, and size of a chart element.

✓ Select the chart element that needs a facelift. To select a chart element, either click it or choose its name on the Chart Elements drop-down.

✓ Format the chart element you selected.

Use one of these methods to format the chart element:

✓ Open a Format dialog box. The dialog box offers commands for formatting the element you selected.

✓ Do the work on your own. For example, to change fonts in the chart element you selected, right-click and choose a font on the shortcut menu. Or go to the Home tab to change font sizes. Or open the drop-down list on the Shape Fill button on the (Chart Tools) Format tab and select a new colour.

Saving a Chart as a Template

Follow these steps to make a template out of a chart:

✓ Save your file to make sure that the chart settings are saved on your computer.

✓ Select your chart.

✓ Go to the (Chart Tools) Design tab.

✓ Click the Save as Template button. You can find this button in the Type group. You will see the Save Chart Template dialog box.

✓ Enter a descriptive name for the template and click the Save button. Include the type of chart you're dealing with in the name. This will help you understand which template you're selecting when the time comes to choose a chart template.

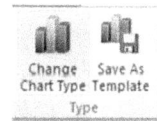

Inserting a picture

✓ Select your chart.

✓ On the (Chart Tools) Format tab, open the Chart Elements drop-down list and choose Plot Area.

✓ Click the Shape Fill button and choose Picture on the drop-down list. You will see the Insert Picture dialog box.

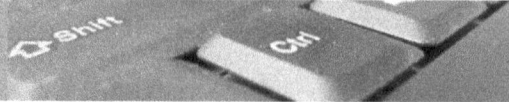

✓ Locate the picture you need and select it. Try to select a light-coloured picture that will serve as a background.

✓ Click the Insert button. The picture lands in your chart.

Annotating a chart

✓ Select your chart and go to the (Chart Tools) Layout tab.

✓ Click the Shapes button, scroll to the Callouts section of the dropdown list, and choose a callout.

✓ Depending on the size of your screen, you may have to click the Insert button to get to the Shapes button.

✓ Drag on your slide to draw the callout shape.

✓ Type the annotation inside the callout shape.

✓ Resize the callout shape as necessary to make it fit with the chart

✓ Drag the yellow diamond on the callout shape to attach the callout to the chart.

SmartArt

this chapter you will learn

- Using Diagrams & shapes in file or document
- Using hybrid layouts with diagrams & Text together

Creating a diagram

After you select a generic diagram in the Choose a SmartArt Graphic dialog box and click OK, the next step is to make the diagram your own by completing these tasks:

❑ **Change the diagram's size and position:** Change the size and position of a diagram to make it fit squarely on your page or slide. See "Changing the Size and Position of a Diagram," later in this chapter.

❑ **Add shapes to (or remove shapes from) the diagram:** Adding a shape involves declaring where to add the shape, promoting or demoting the shape with respect to other shapes, and declaring how the new shape connects to another shape. See "Laying Out the Diagram Shapes" later in this chapter.

❑ **Enter text:** Enter text on each shape, or component, of the diagram. See "Handling the Text on Diagram Shapes" later in this chapter. If you so desire, you can also customize your diagram by taking on some oral of these tasks:

❑ **Changing its overall appearance:** Choose a different colour scheme or 3-D variation for your diagram. See "Choosing a Look for Your Diagram" later in this chapter.

❑ **Changing shapes:** Select a new shape for part of your diagram, change the size of a shape, or assign different colours to shapes to make shapes stand out. See "Changing the Appearance of Diagram Shapes" later in this chapter.

Creating a diagram

Follow these steps to create a diagram:

✓ On the Insert tab, click the SmartArt button. You will see the Choose a SmartArt Graphic dialog box; you can also open the dialog box by clicking the SmartArt Icon in a content placeholder frame.

✓ Select a diagram in the Choose a SmartArt Graphic dialog box. Diagrams are divided into eight categories.

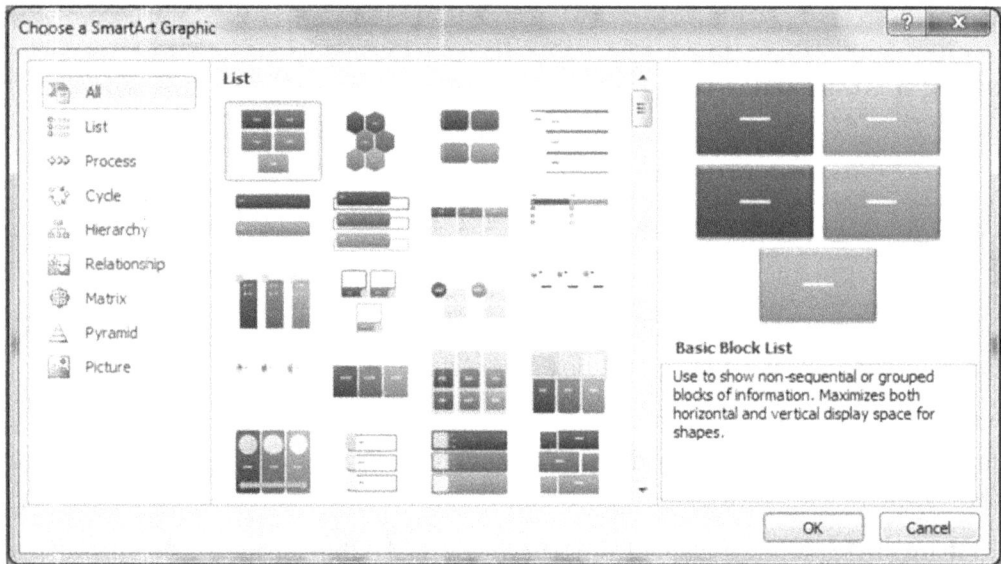

✓ Click your diagram to select it.

✓ Go to the (SmartArt Tools) Design tab.

✓ Open the Layouts gallery (you may have to click the Change Layout button first).You will see a gallery with diagrams of the same type as the diagram you're working with. Select a new diagram or choose More Layouts to open the Choose a SmartArt Graphic dialog box and select a diagram there.

Changing Size and Position of a diagram

To make a diagram fit squarely on a page or slide, you have to change its size and position.

❑ **Resizing a diagram:** Select the diagram, move the pointer over a selection handle on the corner or side, and start dragging after the pointer changes into a two-headed arrow. You can also go to the (SmartArt Tools) Format tab and enter new measurements in the Width and Height boxes. (You may have to click the Size button to see these text boxes, depending on the size of your screen.) ⟷

❑ **Repositioning a diagram:** Select the diagram, move the pointer over its perimeter, and when you see the four-headed arrow, click and start dragging. ✥

Adding shapes to diagrams apart from hierarchy diagrams

Follow these steps to add a shape to a list, process, cycle, relationship, matrix, or pyramid diagram:

✓ In your diagram, select the shape that your new shape will appear before or after.

✓ Choose the Add Shape After or Add Shape Before command. To get to these commands, use one of these methods:

    ✓ On the (SmartArt Tools) Design tab, open the drop-down list on the Add Shape button and choose Add Shape After or Add Shape Before.

    ✓ Right-click the shape you selected, choose Add Shape on the shortcut menu, and then choose Add Shape After or Add Shape Before on the submenu.

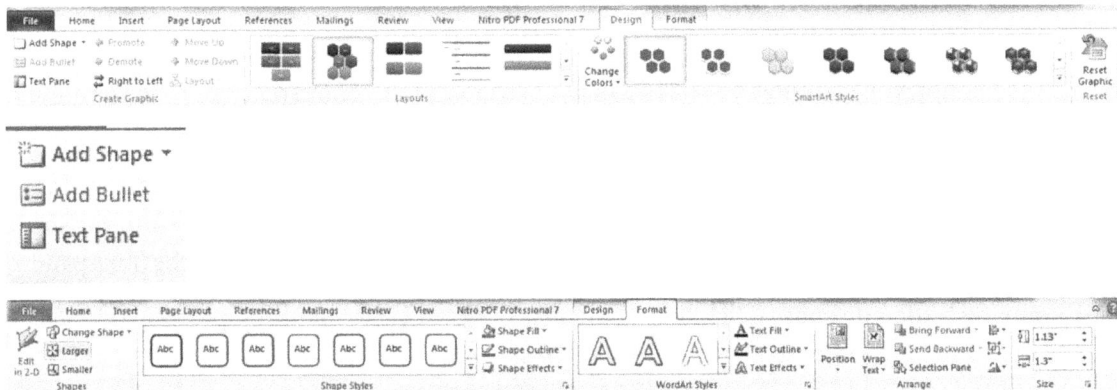

Adding an Organization Chart shape

Besides adding a shape after, before, above, or below a shape, you can add an assistant shape to an Organization Chart diagram. An assistant shape is an intermediary shape between two levels. Follow these steps to add a shape to an Organization Chart diagram:

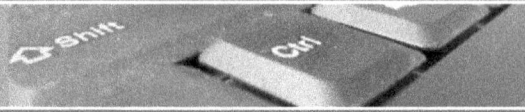

✓ Select the shape to which you will add a new shape.

✓ Choose an Add Shape command.

You can choose Add Shape commands in two ways:

✓ On the (SmartArt Tools) Design tab, open the drop-down list on the Add Shape button and choose an Add Shape command.

✓ Right-click the shape you selected, choose Add Shape on the shortcut menu, and then choose an Add Shape command on the submenu.

Entering text on a diagram shape

Use one of these techniques to enter text on a diagram shape:

✓ Click on the shape and start typing: The words you type appear.

✓ Enter text in the Text pane: Enter the text by typing it in the Text pane

✓ On the (SmartArt Tools) Design tab, click the Text Pane button.

✓ Click the Text Pane button on the diagram. This button is not labeled, but you can find it to the left of the diagram.

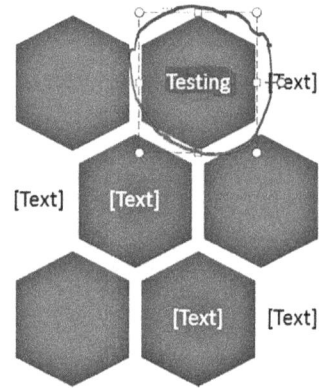

Entering bulleted lists on diagram shapes

Some diagram shapes have built-in bulleted lists, but no matter. Whether a shape is prepared to be bulleted or not, you can enter bullets in a diagram shape. Here are instructions for entering and removing bullets:

❏ **Entering a bulleted list:** Select the shape that needs bullets, and on the (SmartArt Tools) Design tab, click the Add Bullet button. Either enter the bulleted items directly into the shape (pressing Enter as you type each entry) or click the Text Pane button to open the Text pane.

❏ **Removing bulleted items:** Click before the first bulleted entry and keep pressing the Delete key until you have removed all the bulleted items.

Changing a Diagram's direction

✓ Select the diagram.

✓ On the (SmartArt Tools) Design tab, click the Right to Left button. If you don't like what you see, click the button again or click the Undo button.

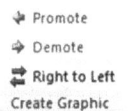

Changing the size of a diagram shape

Select your shape and use one of these methods to enlarge or shrink it:

- ✓ On the (SmartArt Tools) Format tab, click the Larger or Smaller buttons as many times as necessary to make the shape the right size.

- ✓ Move the pointer over a corner selection handle, and when the pointer changes to a two-headed arrow, click and start dragging.

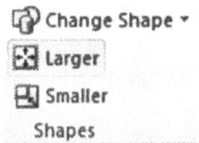

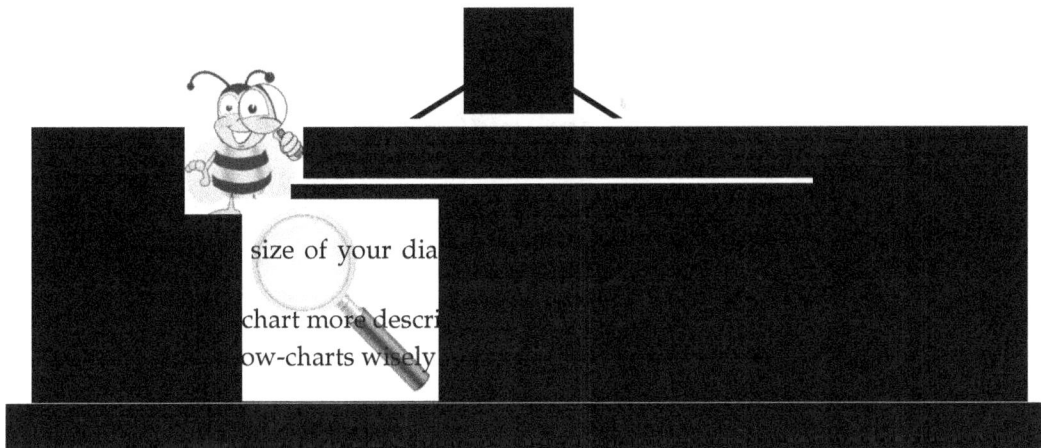

size of your dia

chart more descri

ow-charts wisely

8th Chapter

Drawing Lines & other Shapes

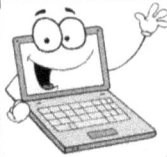

this chapter you will learn

■ Ways to manipulate lines, shapes, text boxes, WordArt images, clip-art images, and graphics

The Basics: Drawing Lines, Arrows, and Shapes

Follow these basic steps to draw a line, arrow, or shape:

✓ Go to the Insert tab.

✓ Click the Shapes button to open the Insert Shapes gallery.

✓ Select a line, arrow, or shape in the Shapes gallery.

✓ Drag on your page, slide, or worksheet. As you drag, the line, arrow, or shape appears.

✓ To alter your line, arrow, or shape—that is, to change its size, colour, or outline—go to the (Drawing Tools) Format tab. This tab offers many commands for manipulating lines and shapes.

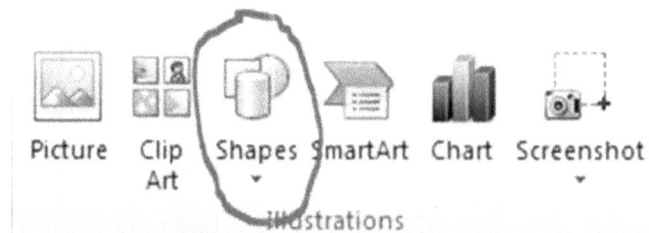

Picture   Clip   Shapes SmartArt   Chart   Screenshot
           Art
                      Illustrations

Handling Lines, Arrows, and Connectors

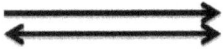

Changing the length and position of a line or arrow

To change anything about a line or arrow, start by clicking to select it. You can tell when a line has been selected because round selection handles appear at either end. Follow these instructions to move a line or adjust its length or angle:

❑ **Changing the angle of a line:** Drag a selection handle up, down, or sideways. A dotted line shows where your line will be when you release the mouse button.

❑ **Changing the length:** Drag a selection handle away from or toward the opposite selection handle.

❑ **Changing the position:** Move the pointer over the line itself and click when you see the four-headed arrow. Then drag the line to a new location.

Changing the appearance of a line, arrow, or connector

What a line looks like is a matter of its colour, its weight (how wide it is), its dash status (it can be filled out or dashed), and its cap (its ends can berounded, square, or flat). To change the appearance of a line, start by selecting it, going to the (Drawing Tools) Format tab, and opening the drop-down list on the Shape Outline button (this button is in the Shape Styles group).

❑ **Colour:** Select a colour on the drop-down list.

❑ **Width:** Choose Weight on the drop-down and then choose a line width on the submenu. You can also choose More Lines on the submenu to open the Format Shape dialog box and change the width there. Enter a setting in points to make the line heavier or thinner.

❑ **Dotted or dashed lines:** Choose Dashes on the drop-down list and then choose an option on the submenu. Again, you can choose More Lines to open the Format Shape dialog box and choose from many dash types and compound lines.

❑ **Line caps:** Click the Shape Styles group button to open the Format Shape dialog box. In the Line Style category, select a cap type (Square, Round, or Flat).

Making the connection

Before you draw the connections, draw the shapes and arrange them on the slide where you want them to be in your diagram. Then follow these steps to connect two shapes with a connector:

✓ Select the two shapes that you want to connect. To select the shapes, hold down the Ctrl key and click each one.

- ✓ On the (Drawing Tools) Format tab, open the Shapes gallery.

- ✓ Under Lines, select the connector that will best fit between the two shapes you want to link together.

- ✓ Move the pointer over a side selection handle on one of the shapes you want to connect. The selection handles turn red.

- ✓ Click and drag the pointer over a selection handle on the other shape, and when you see red selection handles on that shape, release the mouse button. Red, round selection handles appear on the shapes where they're connected. These red handles tell you that the two shapes are connected and will remain connected when you move them.

Handling Rectangles, Ovals, Stars, and Other Shapes

Drawing a shape

Follow these steps to draw a shape:

- ✓ On the Insert tab, click the Shapes button to open the Shapes gallery. You can also insert shapes from the Shapes gallery on the (Drawing Tools) Format tab.

- ✓ Select a shape in the gallery. If you've drawn the shape recently, you may be able to find it at the top of the gallery under Recently Used Shapes.

- ✓ Click and drag slantwise to draw the shape. Hold down the Shift key as you drag if you want the shape to retain its proportions. For example, to draw a circle, select the Oval shape and Hold down the Shift key as you draw.

Changing a shape's size and shape

Selection handles appear on the corners and sides of a shape after you select it. With the selection handles showing, you can change a shape's size and shape:

- ✓ Hold down the Shift key and drag a corner handle to change a shape's size and retain its symmetry.

- ✓ Drag a side, top, or bottom handle to stretch or scrunch a shape.

Choosing a different shape

To exchange one shape for another, select the shape and follow these steps:

- ✓ On the (Drawing Tools) Format tab, click the Edit Shape button.

- ✓ You can find this button in the Insert Shapes group.

✓ Choose Change Shape on the drop-down list.

✓ Select a new shape in the Shapes gallery.

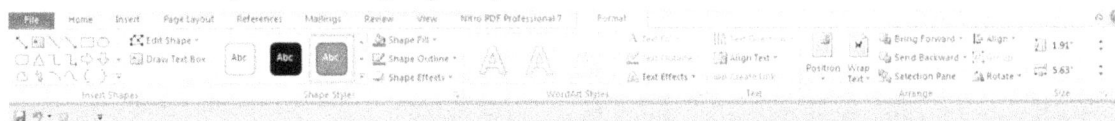

Changing a shape's symmetry

A yellow diamond, sometimes more than one, appears on some shapes. By dragging a diamond, you can change a shape's symmetry.

Follow these instructions to handle text box shapes:

❑ **Entering the text:** Click in the shape and start typing. In Word, you can right-click and choose Add Text if you have trouble typing in the shape.

❑ **Editing the text:** Click in the text and start editing. That's all there is to it. If you have trouble getting inside the shape to edit the text, select the shape, right-click it, and choose Edit Text on the shortcut menu.

❑ **Changing the font, colour, and size of text:** Right-click in the text and choose Font. Then, in the Font dialog box, choose a font, font colour, and a font size for the text.

WordArt for Bending, Spindling, and Mutilating Text

❑ **Allowing the shape to enlarge for text:** You can allow the shape to enlarge and receive more text. Click the Shape Styles group button, and in the Text Box category of the Format Shape dialog box, select the Resize Shape to Fit Text option button.

Creating a WordArt image

Follow these steps to create a WordArt image:

✓ On the Insert tab, click the WordArt button. A drop-down list with WordArt styles appears.

✓ Select a WordArt style.

✓ Enter the text for the image in the WordArt text box.

Editing a WordArt image

On the (Drawing Tools) Format tab, click the Edit Shape button, choose Change Shape, and then select a shape in the Shapes gallery. After the conversion, you usually have to enlarge the shape to accommodate the text. Usually, you have to wrestle with a WordArt image before it comes out right. Select the image, go to the (Drawing Tools) Format tab, and follow the steps:

- ❑ **Editing the words:** Click in the WordArt text box and edit the text there.

- ❑ **Choosing a new WordArt style:** Open the WordArt Styles gallery and select a style. Depending on the size of your screen and which program you're working in, you may have to click the Quick Styles button first

- ❑ **Changing the letters' colour:** Click the Text Fill button and choose a colour on the drop-down list.

- ❑ **Changing the letters' outline:** Click the Text Outline button and make choices to change the letters' outline.

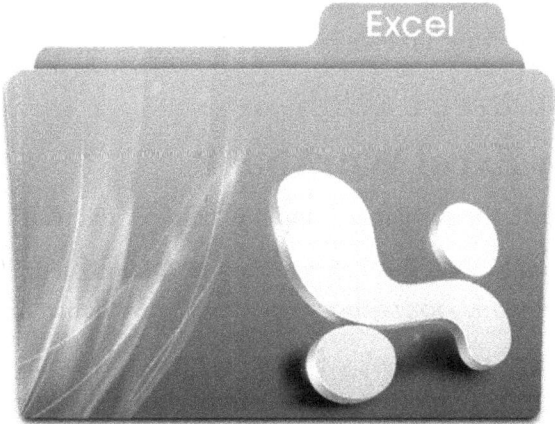

Excel

Welcome to MS Excel

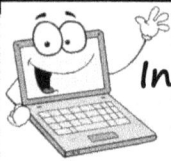

In this chapter you will learn

- Getting started with the Excel screen
- Creating an Excel worksheet
- Formatting & using worksheet
- Selecting text so that you can copy, move, or delete it
- Making custom rules

Creating a New Excel Workbook

Use one of these methods in the Available Templates window to create a workbook:

❑ **Create a blank workbook:** Double-click the Blank Workbook icon. (By pressing Ctrl+N, you can create a new, blank workbook without opening the Available Templates window.)

❑ **Create a workbook from a template:** Use a template on your computer: Click Sample Templates. Templates that you loaded on your computer when you installed Office appear in the window.

❑ **Download a template from Office.com:** Under Office.com Templates, either choose the type of template you want or make sure that your computer is connected to the Internet, enter a search term in the Search box, and click the Start Searching button (or press Enter). Choose a template and click the Download button to download it to your computer.

❑ **Use a template you created (or downloaded earlier from Microsoft):** Click the My Templates icon. The New dialog box appears. Select a template and click OK.

❑ **Select a recently used template:** Click the Recent Templates icon and double-click on a template name.

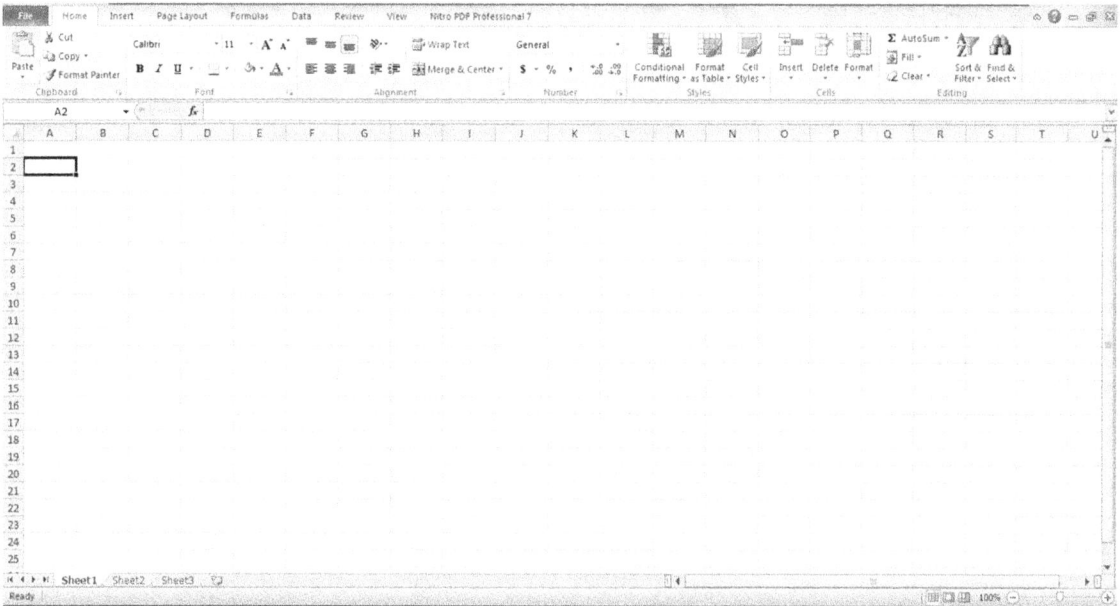

❑ **Recycle another workbook:** If you can use another workbook as the starting point for creating a new one, click the New from Existing icon. In the New from Existing Workbook dialog box, select the workbook and click the Create New button.

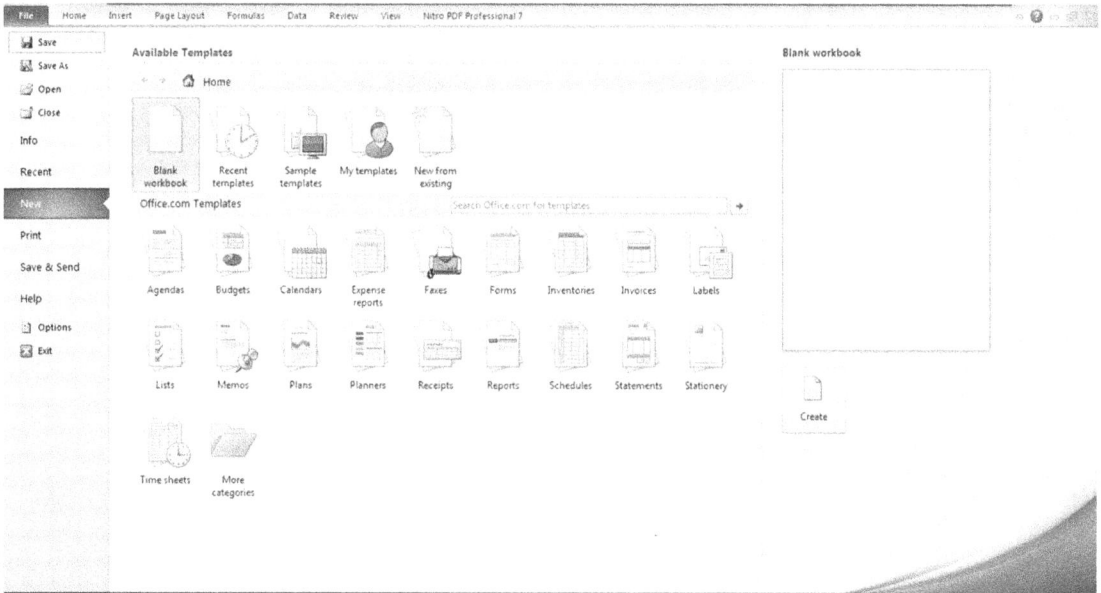

Creating a blank workbook

Rows, columns, and cell addresses

An Excel worksheet has numerous columns and over 1 million rows. The rows are numbered, and columns are labeled A to Z; then AA to AZ; then BA to BZ, and so on. The important thing to remember is that each cell has an address whose name comes from a column letter and a row number. The first cell in row 1 is A1, the second is B1, and so on. You need to enter cell addresses in the formula bar as to tell Excel which numbers to compute. To find a cell's address, either make note of which column and row it lies in, or click the cell and glance at the Formula bar (refer to Figure 1-2). The left side of the Formula bar lists the address of the active cell, the cell that is selected in the worksheet.

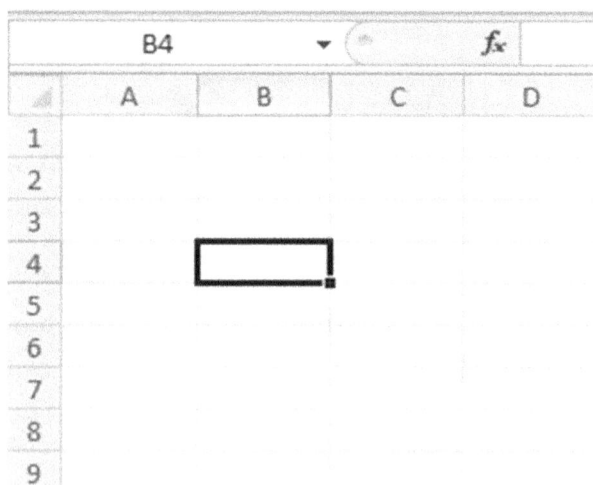

B4		f_x	
A	B	C	D

1			
2			
3			
4			
5			
6			
7			
8			
9			

Workbooks and worksheets

When you create a new Excel file, you open a workbook, a file with three worksheets in it. The worksheets are called Sheet1, Sheet2, and Sheet3 (you can change their names and add more worksheets). To get from worksheet to worksheet, click tabs along the bottom of the Excel window.

Entering Data in a Worksheet

What you can enter in a worksheet cell falls in four categories:

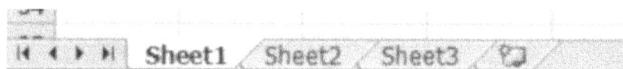

◄ ◄ ► ►|	**Sheet1**	Sheet2	Sheet3	

❑ Text

❑ A value (numeric, date, or time)

❑ A logical value (True or False)

❑ A formula that returns a value, logical value, or text

Procedure

Click the cell where you want to enter the data or text label. The cell you clicked is now the active cell. Glance at the left side of the Formula bar if you're not sure of the address of the cell you're about to enter data in. The Formula bar lists the cell address.

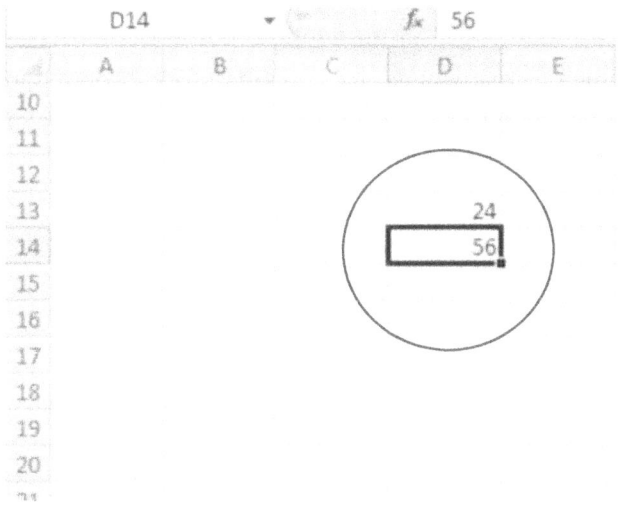

Entering date values

You can enter a date value in a cell in just any format you choose, and Excel understands that you're entering a date. For example, enter a date in any of the following formats and you'll be all right:

m/d/yy 8/31/11

m-d-yyyy 8-31-2011

d-mmm-yy 31-Aug-11

Here are some basic things to remember about entering dates:

❑ **Date formats:** You can quickly apply a format to dates by selecting cells and using one of these methods:

   ✓ On the Home tab, open the Number Format drop-down list and choose Short Date (m/d/yyyy; 8/31/2011) or Long Date (day-of-the-week, month, day, year; Saturday, Aug 31, 2011).

✓ On the Home tab, click the Number group button to open the Number tab of the Format Cells dialog box.

❑ **Current date:** Press Ctrl+; (semicolon) and press Enter to enter the current date.

❑ **Current year's date:** If you don't enter the year as part of the date, Excel assumes that the date you entered is in the current year. For example, if you enter a date in the m/d (8/31) format during the year 2011, Excel enters the date as 8/31/11. As long as the date you want to enter is the current year, you can save a little time when entering dates by not entering the year, as Excel enters it for you.

❑ **Dates on the Formula bar:** No matter which format you use for dates, dates are displayed in the Formula bar in the format that Excel prefers for dates: m/d/yyyy (8/31/2010). How dates are displayed in the worksheet is up to you.

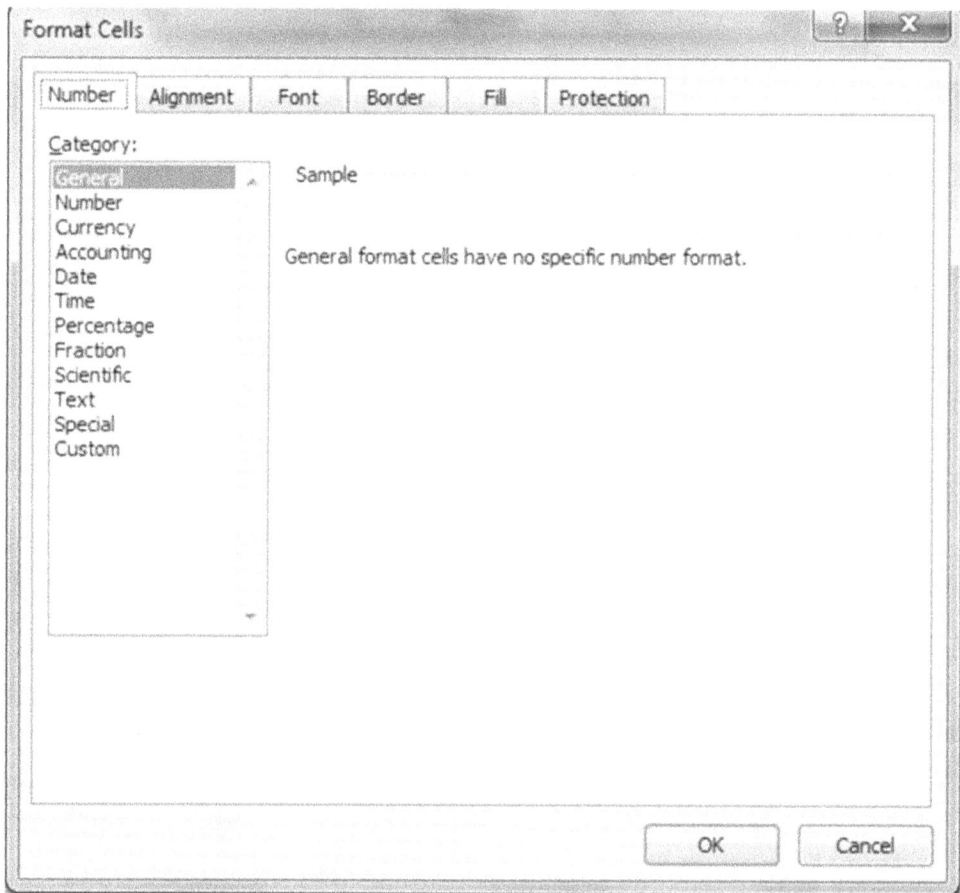

Format cells

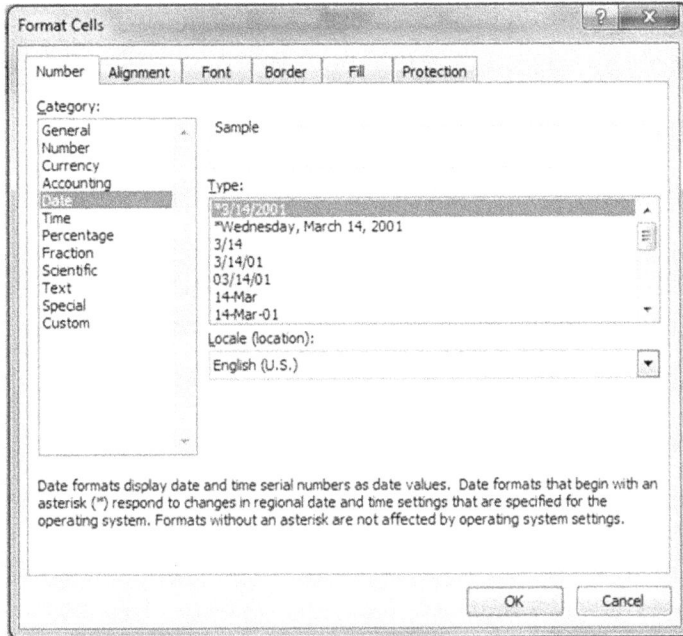

Entering date

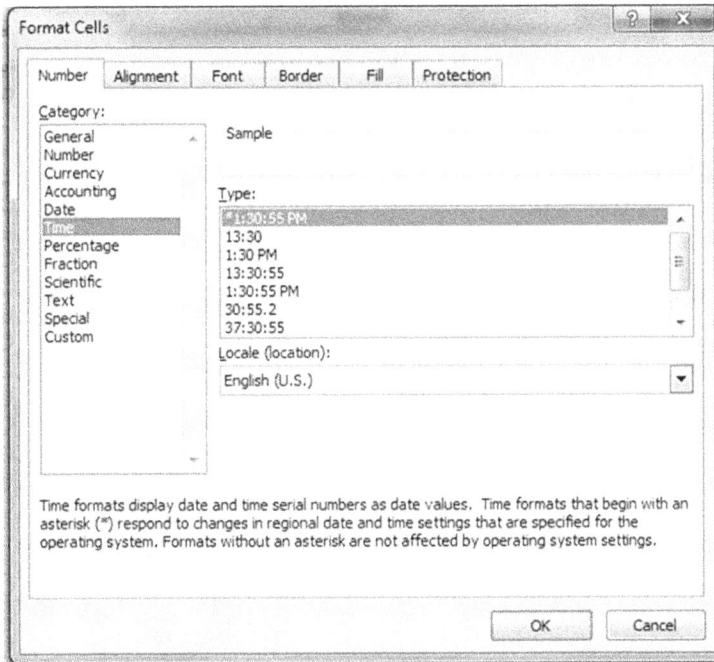

Entering time

- ❑ **20th and 21st century two-digit years:** When it comes to entering two digit years in dates, the digits 30 through 99 belong to the 20th century (1930–1999), but the digits 00 through 29 belong to the 21st century (2000–2029). For example, 8/31/10 refers to August 31, 2010, not August 31,1910.

- ❑ **To enter a date in 1929 or earlier, enter four digits rather than two to describe the year:** 8-31-1929. To enter a date in 2030 or later, enter four digits rather than two: 8-31-2030.

Entering Lists and Serial Data with the AutoFill Command

- ✓ Click the cell that is to be first in the series. For example, if you intend to list the days of the week in consecutive cells, click where the first day is to go.

- ✓ Enter the first number, date, or list item in the series.

- ✓ Move to the adjacent cell and enter the second number, date, or list item in the series. If you want to enter the same number or piece of text in adjacent cells, it isn't necessary to take this step, but Excel needs the first and second items in the case of serial dates and numbers so that it can tell how much to increase or decrease the given amount or time period in each cell. For example, entering 5 and 10 tells Excel to increase the number by 5 each time so that the next serial entry is 15.

- ✓ Select the cell or cells you just entered data in. To select a single cell, click it; to select two, drag over the cells.

- ✓ Click the AutoFill handle and start dragging in the direction in which you want the data series to appear on your worksheet. The AutoFill handle is the little black square in the lower-right corner of the cell or block of cells you selected. Finding it can be difficult. Carefully move the mouse pointer over the lower-right corner of the cell, and when you see the mouse pointer change into a black cross, click and start dragging. As you drag, the serial data appears in a pop-up box, 1.

Formatting Numbers, Dates, and Time Values

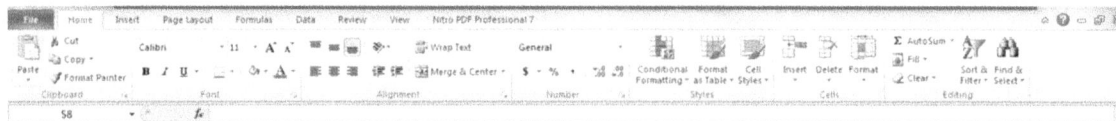

Excel offers five number-formatting buttons on the Home tab — Accounting Number Format, Percent Style, Comma Style, Increase Decimal, and Decrease Decimal. Select cells with numbers in them and click one of these buttons to change how numbers are formatted:

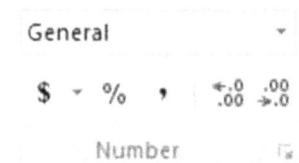

❑ **Accounting Number Format:** Places a dollar sign before the number and gives it two decimal places. You can open the drop-down list on this button and choose a currency symbol apart from the dollar sign. $ ▾

❑ **Percent Style:** Places a percent sign after the number and converts the number to a percentage.

❑ **Comma Style:** Places commas in the number. ❜

❑ **Increase Decimal:** Increases the number of decimal places by one. ⁺.₀₈

❑ **Decrease Decimal:** Decreases the number of decimal places by one. ₊.₀₀

❑ To strip formats from the data in cells, select the cells, go to the Home tab,click the Clear button, and choose Clear Formats. ⬭ Clear ▾

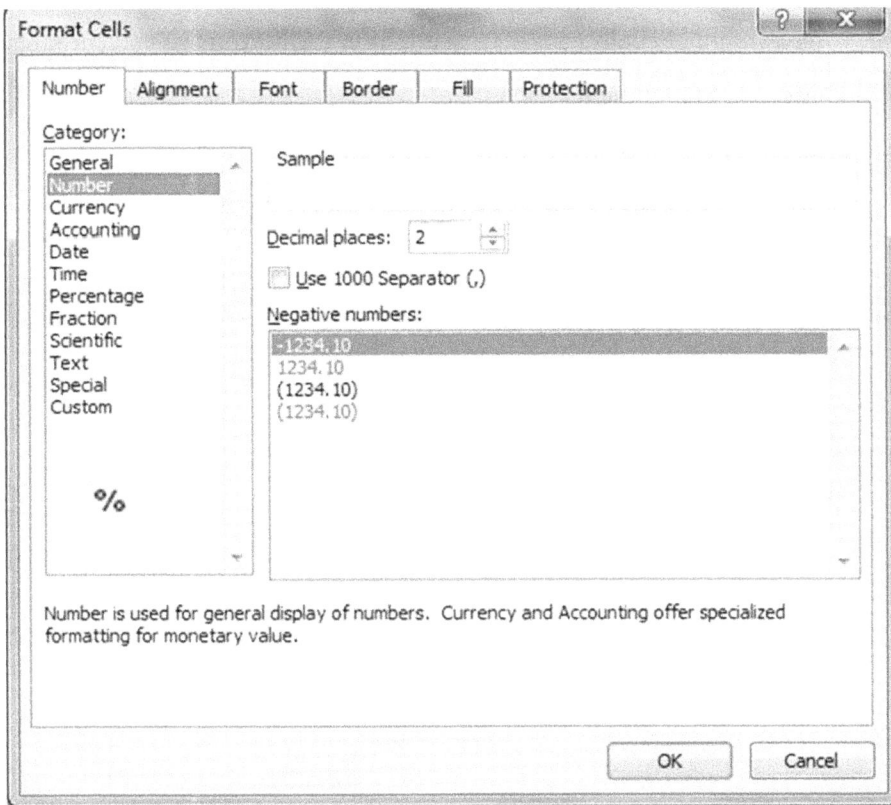

Formatting numbers

Conditional Formats

Select the cells that are candidates for conditional formatting and follow these steps to tell Excel when and how to format the cells:

✓ On the Home tab, click the Conditional Formatting button (you may have to click the Styles button first, depending on the size of your screen).

✓ Choose Highlight Cells Rules or Top/Bottom Rules on the drop-downlist.

You will see a submenu with choices about establishing the rule for whether values in the cells are highlighted or otherwise made more prominent:

❑ **Highlight Cells Rules:** These rules are for calling attention to data if it falls in a numerical or date range, or it's greater or lesser than a specific value. For example, you can highlight cells that are greater.

❑ **Top/Bottom Rules:** These rules are for calling attention to data if it falls within a percentage range relative to all the cells you selected.

For example, you can highlight cells with data that falls in the bottom 50 percent range.

✓ Choose an option on the submenu.

✓ On the left side of the dialog box, establish the rule for flagging data.

✓ On the drop-down list, choose how you want to call attention to the data.

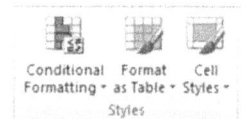

Conditional   Format   Cell
Formatting ▾ as Table ▾ Styles ▾
Styles

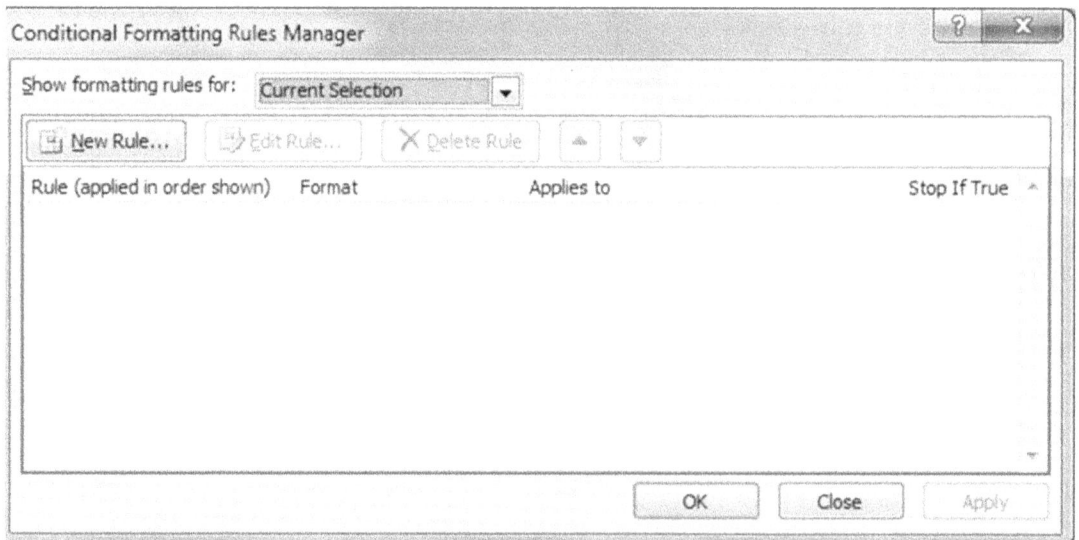

Conditional formatting rules manager

Follow these steps to establish a data-validation rule:

✓ Select the cell or cells that need a rule.

✓ On the Data tab, click the Data Validation button.

✓ On the Allow drop-down list, choose the category of rule you want.

✓ Enter the criteria for the rule.

What the criteria is depends on what rule category you're working in. You can refer to cells in the worksheet by selecting them. To do that, either select them directly or click the Range Selector button and then select them.

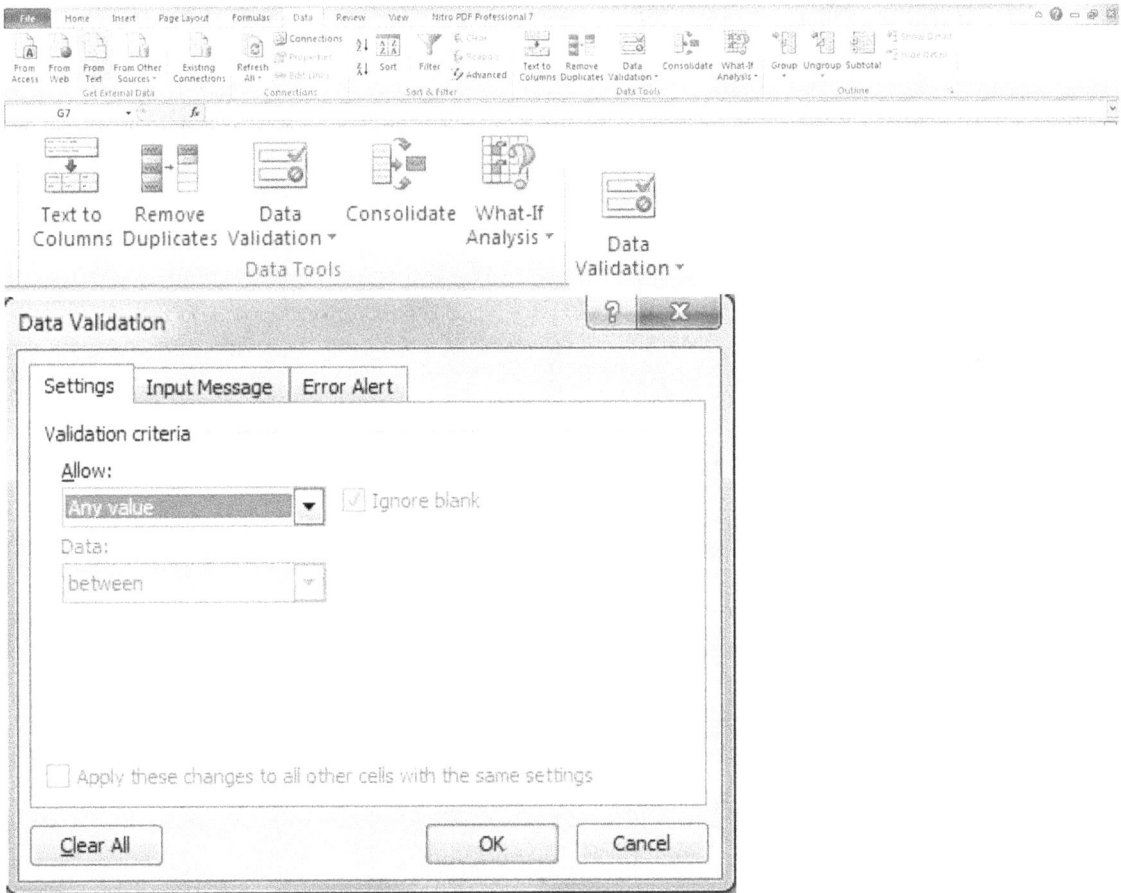

Establishing date validation

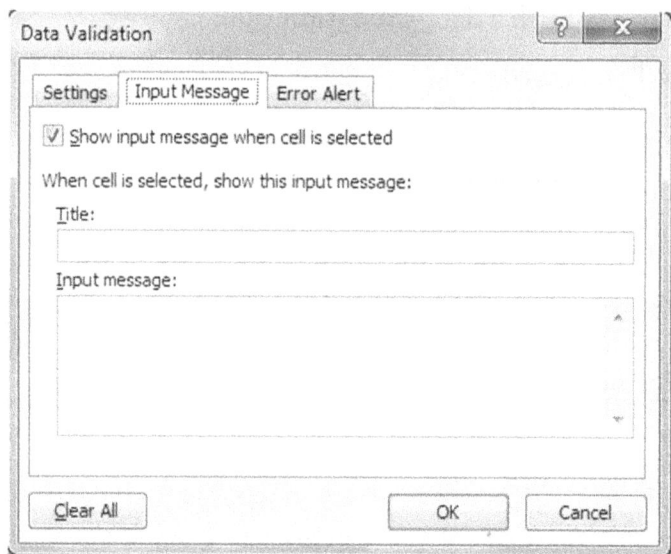

Entering letter and input massage

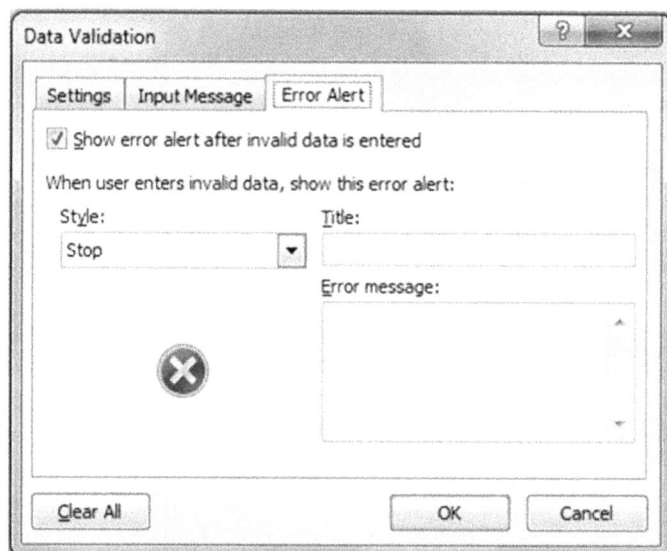

Formatting error alert

✓ On the Input Message tab, enter a title and input message.

✓ On the Error Alert tab, choose a style for the symbol in the Message Alert dialog box, enter a title for the dialog box, and enter a warning message.

✓ Click OK.

To remove data-validation rules from cells, select the cells, go to the Data tab, click the Data Validation button, and on the Settings tab of the Data Validation dialog box, click the Clear All button, and click OK.

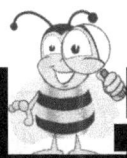

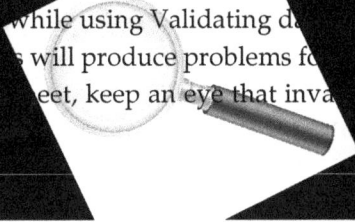

while using Validating d
will produce problems fo
eet, keep an eye that inva

Working on Your Worksheet

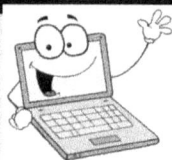

this chapter you will learn

- Editing the worksheet
- Encrypting the document

Editing Worksheet Data

Not everyone enters data correctly the first time. To edit data you entered in a cell, do one of the following:

✓ Double-click the cell. Doing so places the cursor squarely in the cell, where you can start deleting or entering numbers and text.

✓ Click the cell and press F2. This method also lands the cursor in the cell.

✓ Click the cell you want to edit. With this technique, you edit the data on the Formula bar.

Moving in a Worksheet

Keyboard Shortcuts for Worksheets

Press	To Move the Selection
Home	To column A
Ctrl+Home	To cell A1, the first cell in the worksheet
Ctrl+End	To the last cell in the last row with data in it
←, →, ↑, ↓	To the next cell
Ctrl+←, →, ↑, ↓	In one direction toward the nearest cell with data in it or to the first or last cell in the column or row
PgUp or PgDn	Up or down one screen's worth of rows
Ctrl+PgUp or Ctrl+PgDn	Backward or forward through the workbook, from worksheet to worksheet

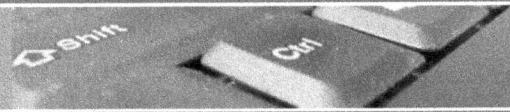

❏ **Scroll bars:** Use the vertical and horizontal scroll bars to move to different areas. Drag the scroll box to cover long distances. To cover long distances very quickly, hold down the Shift key as you drag the scroll box on the vertical scroll bar.

❏ **Scroll wheel on the mouse:** Turn the wheel to quickly scroll up and down.

❏ **Name box:** Enter a cell address in the Name box and press Enter to go to the cell. The Name box is found to the left of the Formula bar.

❏ **Go To command:** On the Home tab, click the Find & Select button, and choose Go To on the drop-down list (or press Ctrl+G or F5). You will see the Go To dialog box. Enter a cell address in the Reference box and click OK. Cell addresses you've already visited with the Go To command are already listed in the dialog box. Click the Special button to open the Go To Special dialog box and visit a formula, comment, or other esoteric item.

❏ **Find command:** On the Home tab, click the Find & Select button, and choose Find on the drop-down list (or press Ctrl+F). Enter the data you seek in the Find What box and click the Find Next button.

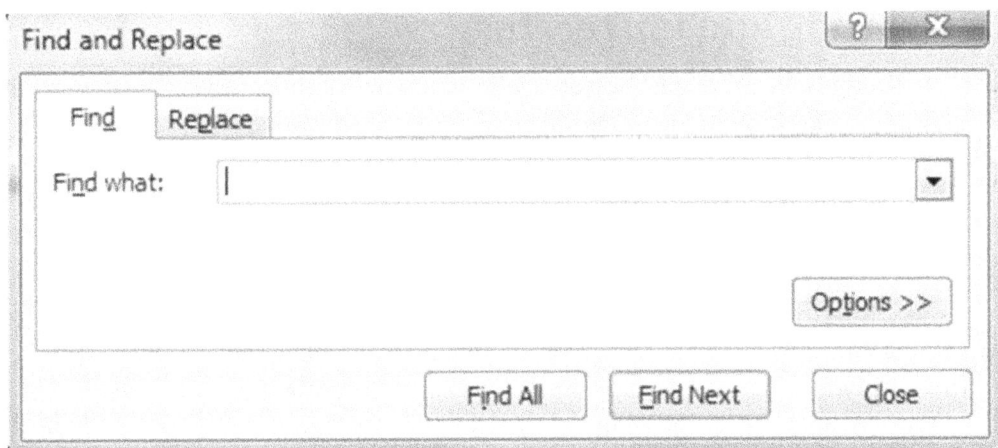

Giving the Split or Freeze Panes command

Follow these steps to split or freeze columns and rows on-screen:

✓ Click the cell directly below the row you want to freeze or split, and click in the column to the right of the column that you want to freeze or split. In other words, click where you want the split to occur.

✓ On the View tab, split or freeze the columns and rows. Go to the View tab and use one of these techniques:

❑ **Splitting:** Click the Split button and then click and drag the split bars ▢ Split to split the screen horizontally or vertically. The other way to split a worksheet is to grab hold of a split bar, the little division markers directly above the vertical scroll bar and directly to the right of the horizontal scroll bar (in the lower-right corner of your screen). You can tell where split bars are because the pointer turns into a double arrow when it's over a split bar.

❑ **Freezing:** Click the Freeze Panes button and choose one of three Freeze options on the drop-down list.

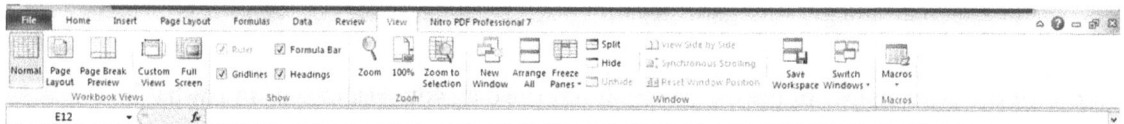

Unsplitting and unfreezing

❑ **Unsplitting:** Click the Split button again; double-click one of the split bars to remove it; or drag a split bar into the top or left side of the worksheet window.

❑ **Unfreezing:** On the View tab, click the Freeze Panes button and choose Unfreeze Panes on the drop-down list.

Hiding columns and rows

❑ **Hiding columns or rows:** Drag over the column letters or row numbers of the columns or rows that you want to hide. Dragging this way selects entire columns or rows. Then go to the Home tab, click the Format button, choose Hide & Unhide, and choose Hide Columns or Hide Rows.

❑ **Unhiding columns and rows:** Select columns to the right and left of the hidden columns, or select rows above and below the hidden rows. To select columns or rows, drag over their letters or numbers. Then go to the Home tab, click the Format button, choose Hide & Unhide, and choose Unhide Columns or Unhide Rows.

Comments for Your Worksheet

❏ **Entering a comment:** Click the cell that deserves the comment, go to the Review tab, and click the New Comment button. Enter your comment in the pop-up box. Click in a different cell when you finish entering your comment.

❏ **Reading a comment:** Move the pointer over the small red triangle and read the comment in the pop-up box.

❏ **Finding comments:** On the Review tab, click the Previous or Next button to go from comment to comment.

❏ **Editing a comment:** On the Review tab, select the cell with the comment, click the Edit Comment button, and edit the comment in the pop-upbox. You can also right-click the cell and choose Edit Comment.

❏ **Deleting comments:** On the Review tab, click a cell with a comment, and then click the Delete button, or right-click the cell and choose Delete Comment. To delete several comments, select them by Ctrl+clicking and then click the Delete button.

❏ **Deleting all comments in a worksheet:** Select all comments and then, on the Review tab, click the Delete button. You can select all comments by clicking the Find & Select button on the Home tab, choosing Go To, and in the Go To dialog box, clicking the Special button and choosingComments in the Go To Special dialog box.

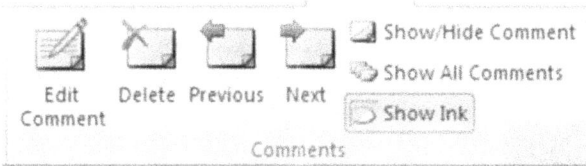

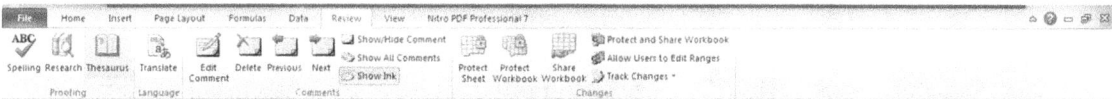

Hiding a worksheet

Follow these instructions to hide and unhide worksheets:

❏ **Hiding a worksheet:** Select the worksheet you want to hide, go to the View tab, and click the Hide button. You can also right-click the worksheet's tab and choose Hide on the shortcut menu. And you can also display the worksheet, go to the Home tab, click the Format button, and choose Hide &Unhide➔Hide Sheet.

☐ 　Hide　**Unhiding a worksheet:** On the View tab, click the Unhide button, select the name
　Unhide　of the worksheet you want to unhide in the Unhide dialog box, and click OK. To
open the Unhide dialog box, you can also right-click any worksheet tab and choose Unhide;
or go to the Home tab.

Protecting a worksheet

✓ Select the worksheet that needs protection.

✓ On the Review tab, click the Protect Sheet button.

✓ Enter a password in the Password to Unprotect Sheet
box if you want only people with the password to be
able to open the worksheet after you protect it.

✓ On the Allow All Users of This Worksheet To list,
select the check box next to the name of each task
that you want to permit others to do. For example,
click the Format Cells check box if you want others
to be able to format cells. Deselect the Select
Locked Cells check box to prevent any changes
from being made to the worksheet. By default,
all worksheet cells are locked, and by preventing
others from selecting locked cells, you effectively
prevent them from editing any cells.

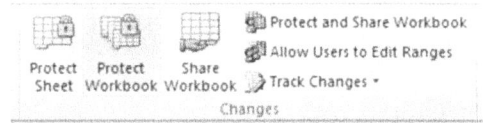

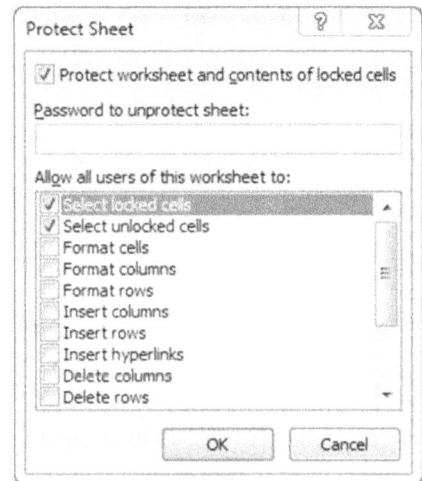

✓ Click OK.

Protection a worksheet

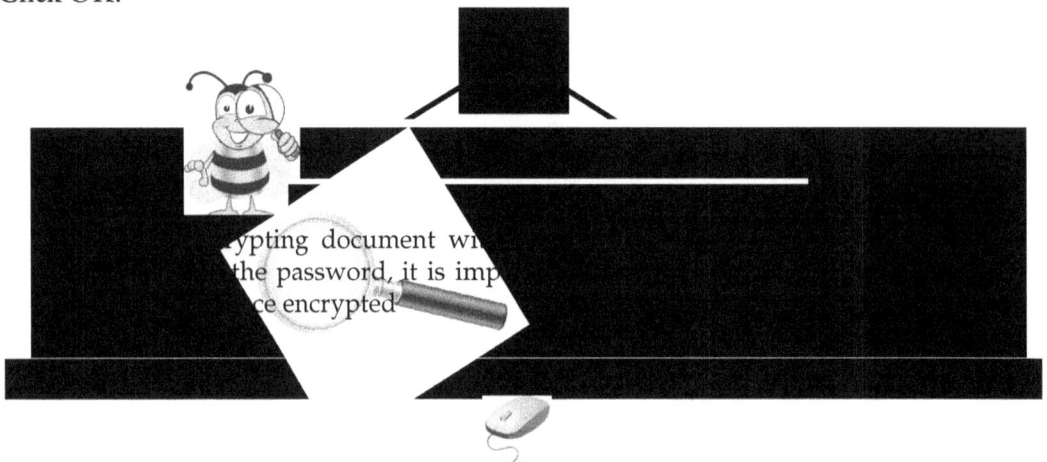

Formulas & Functions

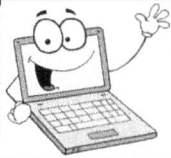

this chapter you will learn

- Using mathematical Formula in the worksheet
- Using Operators in the Worksheet
- Common error messages
- Inserting functions

Referring to cells in formulas

As well as numbers, Excel formulas can refer to the contents of different cells. When a formula refers to a cell, the number in the cell is used to compute the formula. For example, cell A1 contains the number 2; cell A2 contains the number 3; and cell A3 contains the formula =A1+A2. As shown in cell A3, the result of the formula is 5. If I change the number in cell A1 from 2 to 3, the result of the formula in cell A3 (=A1+A2) becomes 6, not 5. When a formula refers to a cell and the number in the cell changes, the result of the formula changes as well.

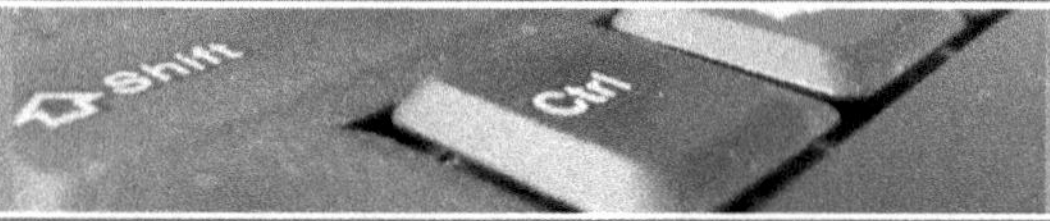

Similarly for Subtraction,

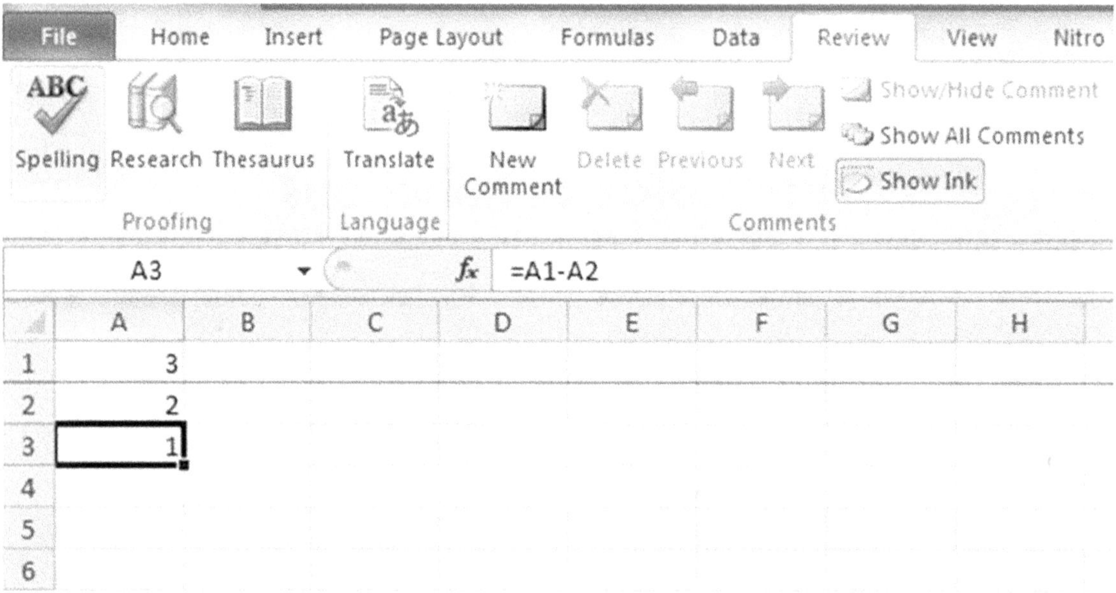

Similarly for Multiplication,

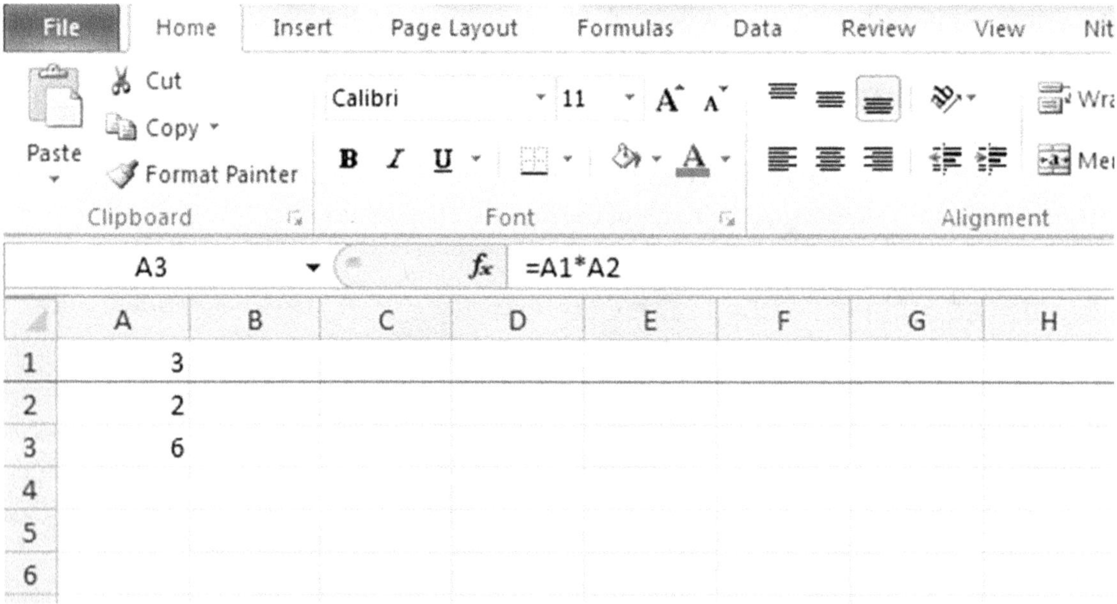

Operators Table

(Most Important! You will need to use these in formulas)

Operator	Example Formula
% (Percent)	=50%
^ (Exponentiation)	=50^2
* (Multiplication)	=E2*4
/ (Division)	=E2/3
+ (Addition)	=F1+F2+F3
– (Subtraction)	=G5–8
= (Equal to)	="Part No."&D4 =C5=4
<> (Not equal to)	=F3<>9
< (Less than)	=B9<E11
<= (Less than or equal to)	=A4<=9
> (Greater than)	=E8>14
>= (Greater than or equal to)	=C3>=D3

Creating a cell range name

Follow these steps to create a cell range name:

✓ Select the cells that you want to name.

✓ On the Formulas tab, click the Define Name button. You see the New Name dialog box.

✓ Enter a descriptive name in the Name box. Names can't begin with a number or include blank spaces.

✓ On the Scope drop-down list, choose Workbook or a worksheet name.

✓ Enter a comment to describe the range name, if you want.

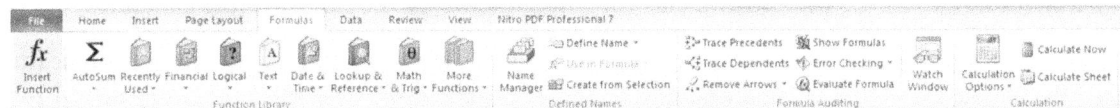

✓ Click OK.

New Name

Name: |

Scope: Workbook

Comment:

Refers to: =Sheet1!A3

OK   Cancel

Name Manager

Define Name ▾
Use in Formula ▾
Create from Selection
Defined Names

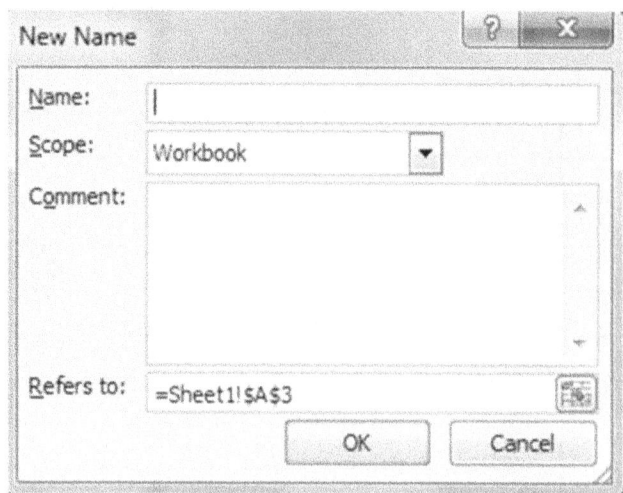

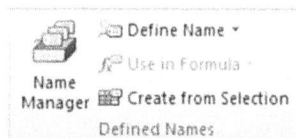

Entering a range name as part of a formula

To include a cell range name in a formula, click in the Formula bar where you want to enter the range name and then use one of these techniques to enter the name:

✓ On the Formulas tab, click the Use in Formula button and choose a cell range name on the drop-down list

✓ Press F3 or click the Use in Formula button and choose Paste Names on the drop-down list.

Managing cell range names

To rename, edit, or delete cell range names, go to the Formulas tab and click the Name Manager button.

✓ **Renaming:** Click the Edit button and enter a new name in the Edit Name dialog box.

✓ **Reassigning cells:** To assign different cells to a range name, click the Edit button. You see the Edit Name dialog box. To enter a new range of cells, either enter the cells' addresses in the Refers To text box or click the Range Selector button (it's to the right of the text box), drag across the cells on your worksheet that you want for the cell range, and click the Cell Selector button again to return to the Edit Name dialog box.

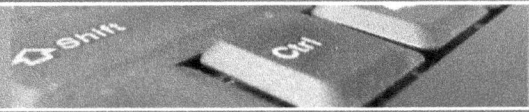

✓ Deleting: Click the Delete button and click OK in the confirmation box.

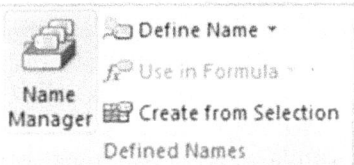

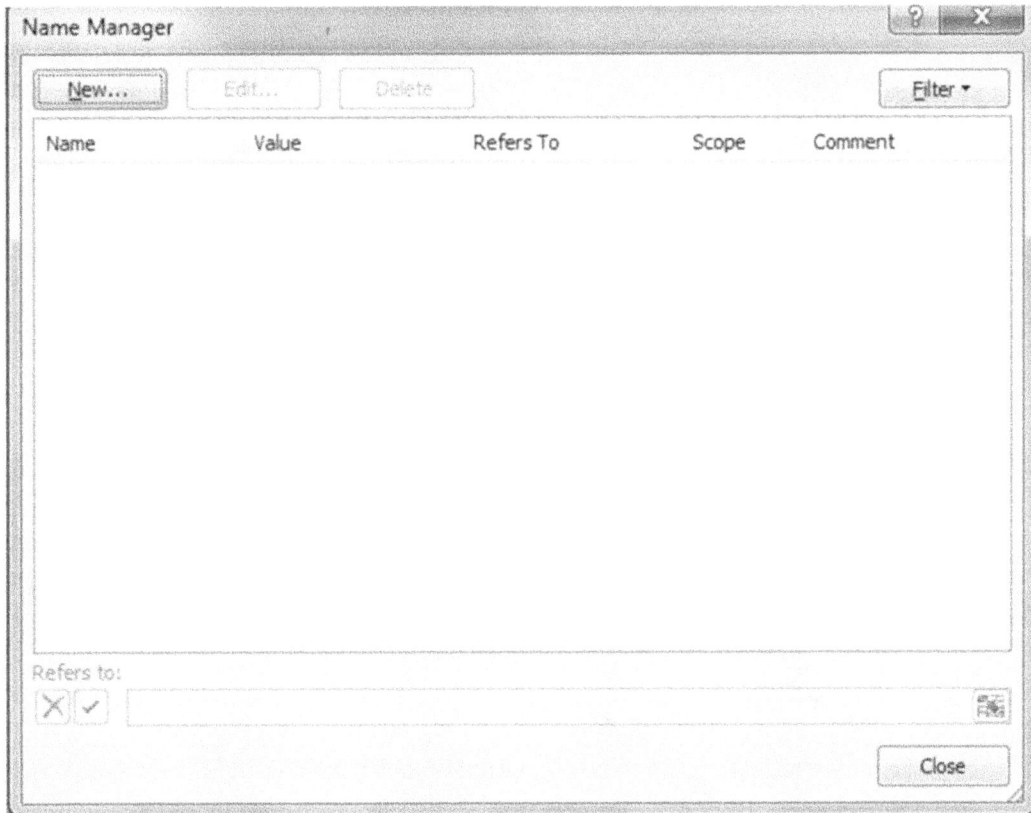

Common Formula Error Messages

Message	Mistake
#DIV/0!	You tried to divide a number by a zero (0) or an empty cell.
#NAME	You used a cell range name in the formula, but the name isn't defined.

Message	Mistake
#N/A	The formula refers to an empty cell, so no data is available for computing the formula. Sometimes people enter N/A in a cell as a place holder to signal the fact that data isn't entered yet. Revise the formula or enter a number or formula in the empty cells.
#NULL	The formula refers to a cell range that Excel can't understand. Make sure that the range is entered correctly.
#NUM	An argument you use in your formula is invalid
#REF	The cell or range of cells that the formula refers to aren't there.
#VALUE	The formula includes a function that was used incorrectly, takes an invalid argument, or is misspelt. Make sure that the function uses the right argument and is spelled correctly.

Common Functions and Their Use

Function	Returns
AVERAGE(number1,number2,...)	The average of the numbers in the cells listed in the arguments.
COUNT(value1,value2,...)	The number of cells that contain the numbers listed in the arguments.
MAX(number1,number2,...)	The largest value in the cells listed in the Arguments.
MIN(number1,number2,...)	The smallest value in the cells listed in the Arguments.
PRODUCT(number1,number2,...)	The product of multiplying the cells listed in the arguments.
STDEV(number1,number2,...)	An estimate of standard deviation based on the sample cells listed in the argument.
STDEVP(number1,number2,...)	An estimate of standard deviation based on the entire sample cells listed in the arguments.
SUM(number1,number2,...)	The total of the numbers in the arguments.
VAR(number1,number2,...)	An estimate of the variance based on the sample cells listed in the arguments.

Function	Returns
VARP(number1,number2,...)	A variance calculation based on all cells listed in the arguments.

Entering a function in a formula

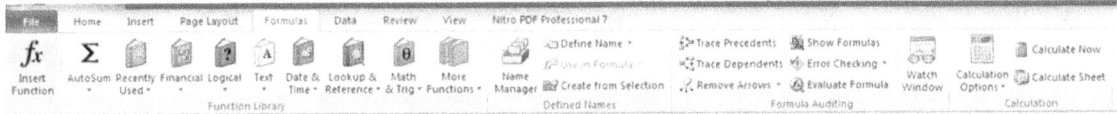

fx
Insert
Function

To enter a function in a formula, you can enter the function name by typingit in the Formula bar, or you can rely on Excel to enter it for you. Enter function names yourself if you're well acquainted with a function and comfortable using it.

No matter how you want to enter a function as part of a formula, start this way:

✓ Select the cell where you want to enter the formula.

✓ In the Formula bar, type an equals sign (=). Be sure to start every formula by entering an equals sign (=). Without it, Excel thinks you're entering text or a numbering the cell.

✓ Start constructing your formula, and when you come to the place where you want to enter the function, type the function's name.

Excel's help in entering a function as part of a formula:

On the Formulas tab, tell Excel which function you want to use.

You can do that with one of these techniques:

❑ **Click a Function Library button:** Click the button whose name describes what kind of function you want and choose the function's name on the drop-down list. You can click the Financial, Logical, Text, Date & Time, Lookup & Reference, Math & Trig, or More Functions buttons.

❑ **Click the Recently Used button: Click** this button and choose the name of a function you used recently.

❑ **Click the Insert Function button:** Clicking this button opens the Insert Function dialog box. Find and choose the name of a function. You can search for functions or choose a category and then scroll the names until you find the function you want.

❑ Enter arguments in the spaces provided by the Function Arguments dialog box. To enter cell references or ranges, you can click or select cells in your worksheet. If necessary, click the Range Selector button (you can find it to the right of an argument text box) to shrink the Function

Arguments dialog box and get a better look at your worksheet.

❏ Click OK when you finish entering arguments for your function. I hope you didn't have to argue too strenuously with the Function Arguments dialog box.

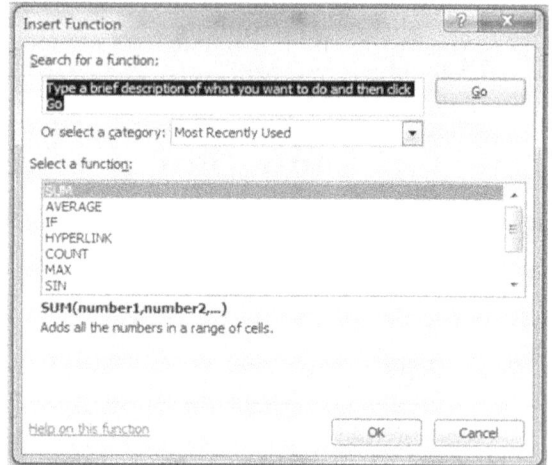

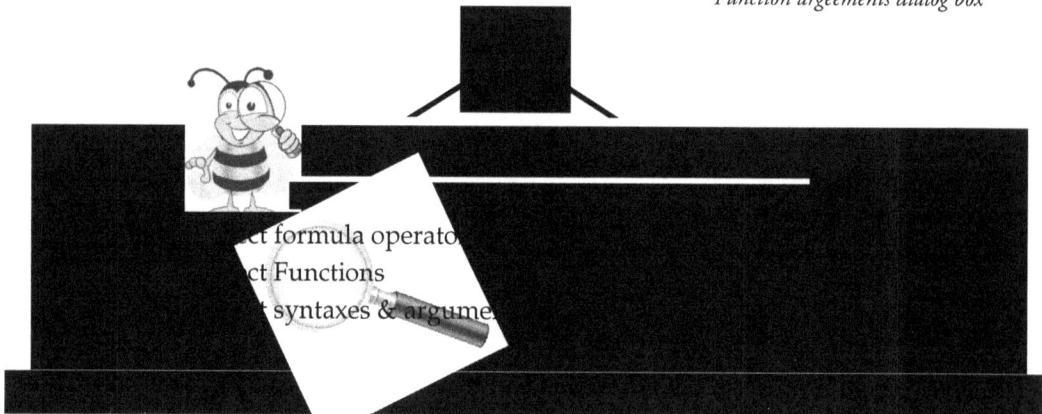

Function argeements dialog box

formula operato
Functions
syntaxes & argume

STUDENT DEVELOPMENT/LEARNING
(छात्र विकास/लर्निंग)

JOKES
(हास्य)

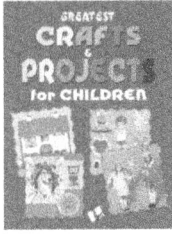
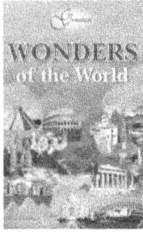
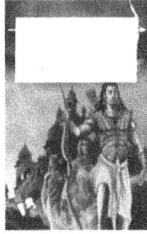
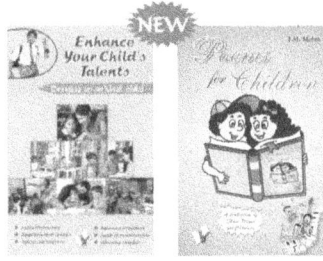
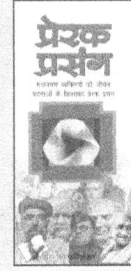
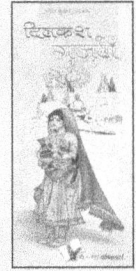

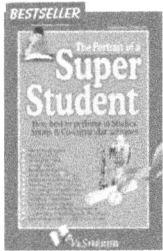
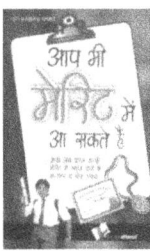
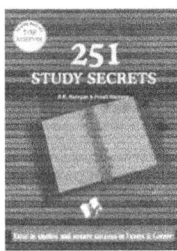
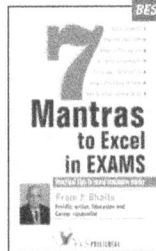
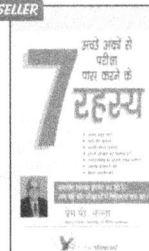
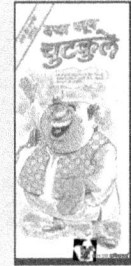
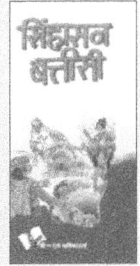

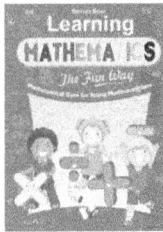
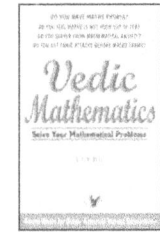
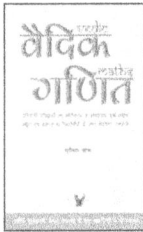
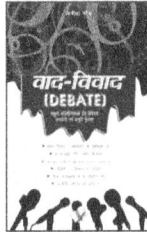
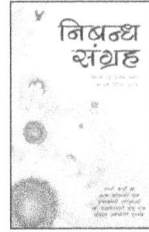
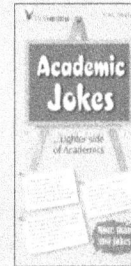
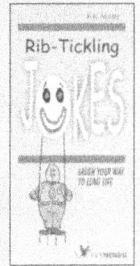

MAGIC & FACT (जादू एवं तथ्य)

MUSIC (संगीत)

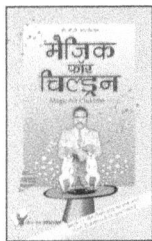
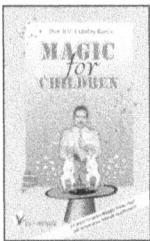
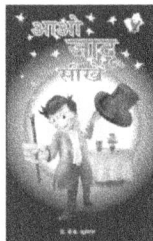
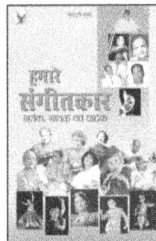
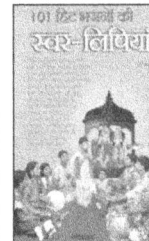
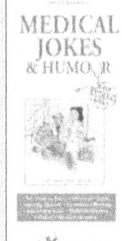
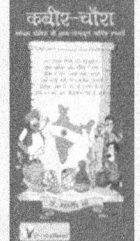

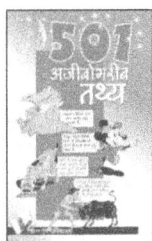
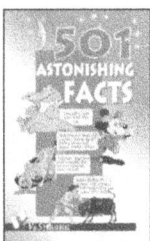
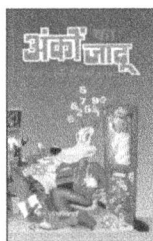

COMPUTER

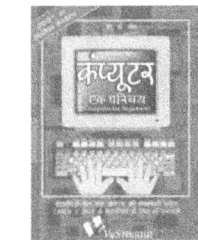
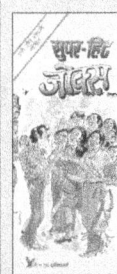
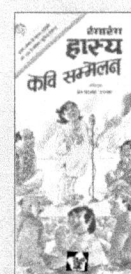
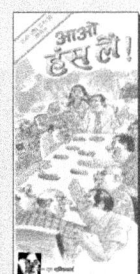

Quiz Books
(प्रश्नोत्तरी की पुस्तकें)

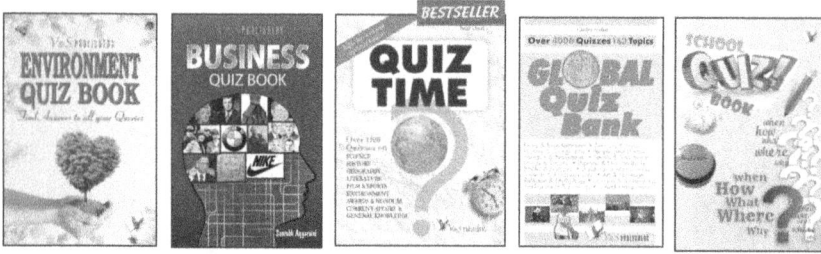

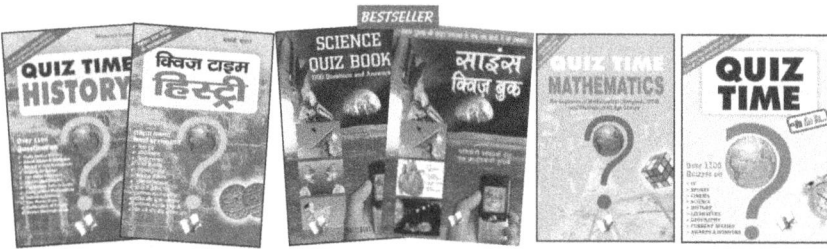

MYSTERIES
(रहस्य)

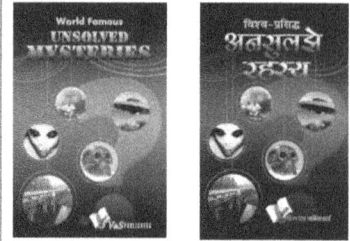

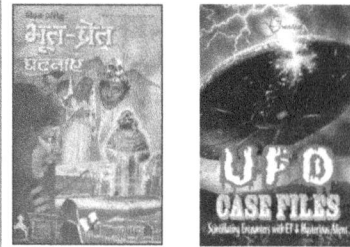

DRAWING BOOKS (ड्राइंग बुक्स)

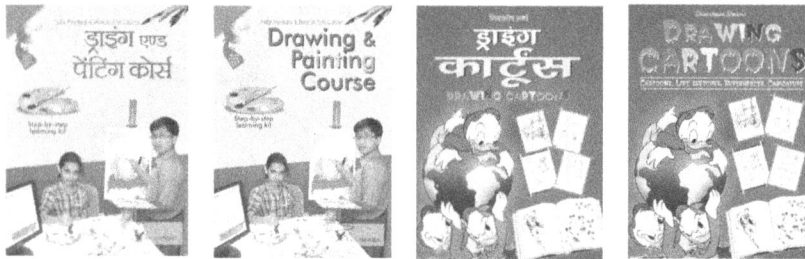

QUOTES/SAYINGS (उद्धरण/सूक्तियाँ)

BIOGRAPHIES (आत्म कथाएँ)

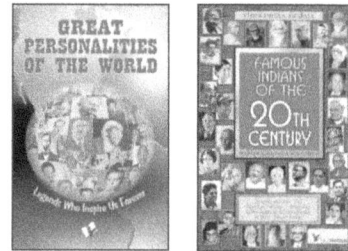

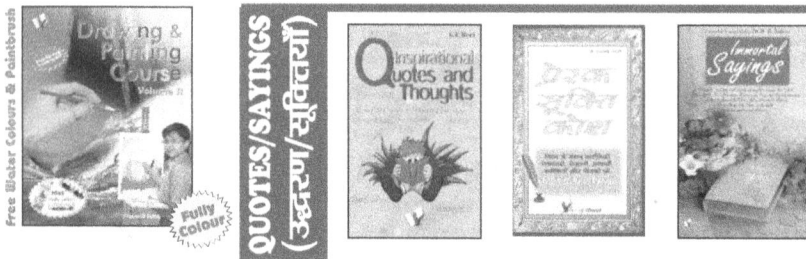

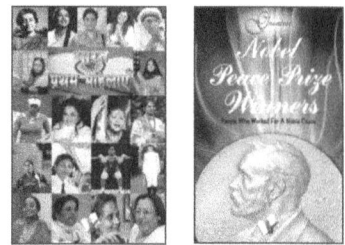

PUZZLES (पहेलियां)

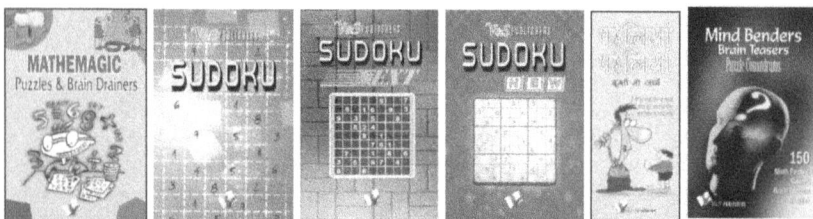

ACTIVITIES BOOK (एक्टिविटीज बुक)

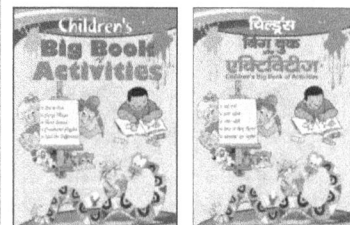

www.ingramcontent.com/pod-product-compliance
Lightning Source LLC
Chambersburg PA
CBHW081420270326
41931CB00015B/3347